EAT FOR STRENGTH

A Vegetarian Cookbook

Oil-Free edition

BLESSED ART THOU, O LAND,
WHEN THY PRINCES **EAT FOR STRENGTH**
AND NOT FOR DRUNKENNESS   Ecclesiastes 10:17

By

Agatha M. Thrash, M.D.

New Lifestyle Books
Route 1, Box 441
Seale, AL 36875

Printed by
Edwards Brothers, Inc.
Lillington, North Carolina

ISBN: 0-942658-01-9

PREFACE

For several years requests have been coming in to prepare a set of recipes and menus for those who want a very simple dietary. Most of these individuals have normal health and are eating a regular vegetarian diet. Some of these, however, have special health needs, such as heart disease, cancer, arthritis, diabetes, or other conditions of accelerated aging. EAT FOR STRENGTH, OIL FREE EDITION, should be helpful for those who desire the advantages of a simple vegetarian dietary.

In preparing this cookbook, a strong effort was made to keep individual dishes unconcentrated and uncomplicated. We believe that the resulting recipes are healthful and will appeal to the educated palate of those who appreciate the natural goodness of food and who desire to attain a high level of healthfulness.

Although this cookbook is designed for those who want to avoid free oils, the cook may desire to use some oil or sweetening, an additional or substitute ingredient, or another flavoring or seasoning. To do so will not spoil the dish. We recommend, however, that complex mixtures be avoided, that pungent flavors be used lightly, and that any concentrated or refined food be included only sparingly. In addition to oil, concentrated and refined foods include salt, sugar, nuts, wheat germ, food yeast, soy milk powder, etc. If a food item has been separated from other parts of the original food it is usually concentrated, or rich in certain elements, and should be used with the thought in mind that the biochemical systems of the body will be put to the stretch to accommodate the rich item. Recipes should not be made rich with **any** nutrient-refined carbohydrates, oils, proteins, vitamins, or minerals. These principles will assist in educating the appetite for a more healthful dietary.

Most of the recipes in EAT FOR STRENGTH, OIL FREE EDITION, can be used by those who need either a completely oil free diet or simply the absence of free fats. To make certain recipes acceptable for completely oil free diets, nuts, seeds, coconut, or wheat germ must be omitted. There are some recipes, however, that contain nuts, seeds, olives, or avocados as an essential ingredient. These recipes must be avoided by those who want a completely oil free diet. May you enjoy a higher level of personal production as you simplify your diet.

CONTENTS

Abbreviations

c. .... cup
gms. .... grams
lb. .... pound
mg. ....milligrams
pkg. .... package
qt. .... quart
t. .... teaspoon
T. ....tablespoon
#2 can .... 2$\frac{1}{2}$ cups

I. BREADS

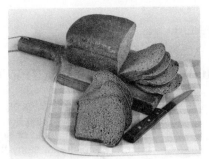

I. BREADS

HOW TO MAKE A RECIPE TURN OUT RIGHT

1. Read recipe carefully, every word of it!
2. Before you begin mixing do whatever special job needs to be done, such as chopping nuts or sifting flour.
3. If there are pictures, study them closely.
4. Turn heat to correct temperature if preheated oven is needed.
5. Get ingredients together on deck. Collect utensils.
6. Measure exactly. It may make a difference.
7. Follow every step exactly as directed.
8. Bake or cook exactly as directed.
9. Cool, or serve at once, or store as directed in recipe.
10. Keep working area orderly throughout procedure.

THE STAFF OF LIFE

The real staff of life is bread, our most important food. Breads are of two types, 1) raised, leavened, or light breads and, 2) unleavened or quick breads. Raised breads are made by some agent able to produce bubbles of gas. We will present leavened breads raised only with yeast, since all baking sodas and baking powders either leave residues in the breads that injure the body, or they damage the grains during the cooking process, making them less nourishing. Yeast used as a leavening does not damage the grain. There are some volatile substances left in the bread after the fermentation process that will completely evaporate after 1–3 days. Yeast bread is much more healthful a few days after baking. The conditioning of the crumb proceeds during the first three days, making the bread more digestible and more easily cut.

Using quick breads freely has many advantages. These breads are simple and quick to make. The long, slow baking of such quick breads as crackers contributes to their digestibility as the starches are dextrinized by the action of heat and water.

A LIFE SYLE OF REGULARITY

A lifestyle of regularity and abstemiousness is strengthening to both mind and body. The cause of a nervous breakdown is often believed to be overwork, whereas the actual cause is too much food eaten at irregular periods, inattention to proper rest and exercise, and often a stimulating lifestyle that taxes the nervous system. The biochemistry of the brain is such that throughout the day there are changes that meet the need of the hour. By carefully cooperating with these changes one can bring about the most favorable functioning of the nervous system. Humans are designed so that they function best if they arise at the same early hour each day, put all major functions such as meals, exercise periods, and study periods, on the same schedule, and go to bed daily at the same hour. This is spoken of as the **Circadian Rhythm**. The digestive system functions best and the most good is obtained from the food eaten if this pattern of cooperating with nature is maintained. It is not normal to be nervous or sick. Proper attention to nature's laws can prevent much ill health that is considered to be unavoidable providential outworkings.

I. BREADS

BAKING THE LOAVES

The temperature should not be so hot as to overcook the outside of the loaf before the inside is cooked. Preheat the oven for 5 minutes at 400°. The bread will rise for the first 10 minutes and by then will have sufficient crust to hold it firm. Loaves need to be small enough that the loaf may be well baked in 45 minutes. A well baked loaf may be lifted from the pan and placed on the palm without burning it, as the moisture is evaporated. Yeast bread should be "light and dry." "Light" is a word having to do with the bubbles made in the dough, and not to the weight of the loaf. Rolls can rise lighter than loaves and still not be in danger of falling.

WARTIME FOOD

During the war some interesting articles came from England on the subject of the importance of bread for the nerves, general health, and especially for the heart. Many men became interested in baking at that time, since there was little opportunity to spend leisure hours away from home. Everyone remembers that during the war the health of the English people improved. The shortage of sugar, the custom of growing a "victory garden," and especially the making of their own bread from whole grains (white grains were not available) all contributed to this improvement.

Bread constitutes one of the most important articles of diet. It should never be omitted from the dietary as it furnishes food elements almost impossible to replace elsewhere. The whole grains contain the following nutrients and trace elements.

Carbohydrates	Phosphorus	Manganese
Protein	Iron	Copper
Fatty Acids	Zinc	Sulphur
Magnesium	Potassium	Iodine
Calcium	Silver	Fluorine
Chlorine	Vitamin E	Pyridoxine
Sodium	Choline	Pantothenic Acid
Silicon	Folic Acid	Niacin
Boron	Inositol	Riboflavin
Barium	Biotin	Thiamine

TIPS FOR SUCCESS IN BREAD MAKING

Don't start a batch of bread until you have read the recipe all the way through, know that you have the proper ingredients or suitable substitutes, and understand the mixing method.

If you are just learning to bake, try a simple basic recipe first, such as **Whole Wheat Bread**.

I. BREADS

GENERAL INSTRUCTIONS

Use only the freshest and best quality of flours. Old flour may not rise. The gluten content of hard wheat flour makes it best for bread making. A mixture of two or three flours is quite nutritious, as the elements of one will supplement deficient elements of another. Breads made from mixtures of two or three grains should be used alternately with single grain breads for best nutrition. To avoid a "complex mixture," do not mix a large number of grains in one loaf.

Keep the temperature right. An off-flavor develops in bread that is allowed to get too warm. Too cool a temperature prolongs the rising. Yeast plants grow best at a temperature of 80°.

Salt and fat both retard the growth of the yeast and preferably should not be added to a yeast mixture until it has grown strong and lively by feeding on sugar and starch. Too much sugar retards the action of the yeast. Sweet breads should have the extra honey added after the yeast is growing well.

Develop the gluten of wheat flour in the batter by beating thoroughly or squeezing between fingers before adding other flours which have no gluten. Gluten toughens on beating, enabling it to hold air bubbles better.

When the dough is ready to mold into loaves, flour your hands and the pans well. Form the dough into a smooth ball or loaf, and tuck it in so that the edges touch the sides of the pan, snugly and smoothly.

Always preheat the oven before the bread is ready to go in. It is a good idea to turn it on when you start molding the loaves as this warms the kitchen and helps the bread to rise quickly. Five minutes preheating is minimal.

When dough is doubled in bulk and ready to bake, a slight indentation made with the finger will remain rather than springing back up. If in doubt, it is better to be "a little on the green side" rather than over-raised.

The loaves should be small and thoroughly baked. No taint of sourness should be present in the bread when the loaf is cut. Allow 12 to 36 hours after baking before eating.

Brushing the crust of the loaf with oil will give a tender crust but adds more oil to an already overfatted diet. Don't cover bread while it is cooling, except with a towel, as it causes a soft, slightly damp crust.

The addition of soy flour gives a more moist product that keeps fresh a long time. There are two general types of soy flour: high-fat and low-fat. The low-fat has a higher percentage of protein than the high-fat and also keeps better. Both are of a high order of digestibility and are free from any objectionable "bean" flavor.

Flours grow stale and rancid on aging. For this reason it is well to keep all grains, whether whole or ground, refrigerated or frozen during storage.

Bold Print indicates items listed in the INDEX

GOOD BREAD

Start with good materials. The utensils and equipment should be sturdy, well cleaned, and not of toxic material. The flours, if naturally balanced as they come from the Creator, will support the life of molds and weevils. Polishing and milling, even if followed by "enriching," actually impoverish the grain.

Stale flour will not rise well and does not have a good flavor. Vitality has been lost.

Allow no harmful additives such as preservatives or conditioners.

Keep the yeast fresh and constantly replenished for best results. It is not necessary to change to new yeast types when genuine baker's yeast is being used.

Find the best recipe possible and after careful testing, value it forever.

Follow the recipe. Even the best recipe is worth little if it is not faithfully followed.

Constant care after baking. Allow to cool, store properly, but keep stock continually changed.

Eat with thanksgiving.

Share what you have with others.

Eat "all of it," chewing well.

GOOD RELIGION

Protect virture in the same way one protects fine grains. Keep out eroding influences, and a virtuous life will make a strong character that will exert a life-giving influence on all.

Develop the good qualities by proper associations and daily use.

Good religion needs no paganism, pomp, or human qualities to make it effective and life-giving.

Faith must be constantly exercised. It should be always fresh and new. Even though not novel, or different in essence today than yesterday, it will be effective in elevating and ennobling the soul.

The recipe for life is the Bible. Each word or spirit must be carefully tested by the Bible. Treasure the Bible as the priceless Word of God.

It is essential to actually observe the truths of the Bible, the Ten Commandments. Mere knowledge of the Word is worth little.

A justification experience is not adequate for salvation unless carefully preserved by a sanctification process.

"A merry heart doeth good like a medicine."

Light hoarded soon becomes darkness. We must constantly witness in order to remain alive.

Just as the Passover Lamb had to be entirely eaten and assimilated to be effective, so we must use and assimilate all parts of the grain in order to receive the full benefit.

I. BREADS

THE SPICE OF LIFE

As in all other foods, VARIETY is the watchword in breads. As good as whole wheat is, it is not best to serve it as a steady diet. Rye, corn, oats, and other grains should be used to make breads. Not all bread should be yeast bread, but health will be better, and interest in meals higher if the quick breads are used often, especially crackers, which require thorough chewing.

Variety should also extend to the baking method. While yeast raised breads may be considered quite healthful, it is not wise to use it exculsively or perhaps at every meal served. Some meals should be planned so that yeast leavening is not used. Baker's yeast is capable of elevating the uric acid level in the blood if used largely. While most people will not use bread in sufficient quantity to affect the uric acid level, it would seem wise to use this additional precaution to insure the most healthful possible meals for the family. Some individuals are especially prone to develop gout, and any practice that will raise the uric acid level would be undesirable. For more discussion on this subject see the section on "DAIRY PRODUCT SUBSTITUTES."

BREAD STICKING TO PANS

To prevent sticking to pans there are several directions to investigate. Several new materials for baking dishes and pans seem to be safe. These are of the Teflon type. Sometimes a light sprinkle of corn meal, flour, bran, or oatmeal can be used to prevent sticking. Use your ingenuity to arrive at a satisfactory practice. Some bakers line their pans with wet wrapping paper.

When flour is mixed with water and kneaded, the gluten of the wheat becomes very elastic and adherent. This quality enables it to hold the gas bubbles formed by the yeast, making the bread light and porous. Wheat contains the most tenacious gluten of any grain. Rye contains a small quantity of strong gluten.

A loaf of bread is approximately three-fourths air. Of the one-third left, about thirty-eight per cent is water; fifty per cent is carbohydrate. About ten per cent is protein, almost half the percentage present in beef. In making whole wheat bread, the dough should be about as sticky as can be handled. If the dough gets too soft, however, it will not have a good grain, and may have a harder crust than when properly mixed. White bread dough can be quite stiff, as it does not carry the heavy freight of vitamins and minerals that the whole wheat flour carries. Salt and shortening often retard the action of yeast, and should be added after yeast growth is established if used at all.

Bold Print indicates items listed in the INDEX

I. BREADS

COMMON DEFECTS OF BREAD AND POSSIBLE CAUSES

1. SOUR TASTE
   a. Water too warm.
   b. Period of rising too long, especially in whole grain breads which will not rise as light as white breads.
   c. Temperature too high while rising.
   d. Poor yeast.

2. DRY OR CRUMBLEY
   a. Too much flour in dough.
   b. Over-baking.

3. HEAVINESS
   a. Unevenness of temperature while rising.
   b. Insufficient kneading.
   c. Old flour.
   d. Old yeast.

4. CRACKS IN CRUST
   a. Cooling in a draft.
   b. Baking before sufficiently light.
   c. Oven too hot at first.

5. TOO THICK A CRUST
   a. Oven too slow.
   b. Baked too long.
   c. Excess of salt.

6. DARK PATCHES OR STREAKS
   a. Poor materials.
   b. Shortening added to flour before liquid, thus allowing flour particles to become coated with fat before they had mixed evenly with the liquid.

7. SOGGINESS
   a. Too much liquid.
   b. Insufficient baking.
   c. Cooling in airtight container.

8. ILL-SHAPED LOAF
   a. Not molded well originally.
   b. Too large a loaf for the pan.
   c. Rising period too long.
   d. Failure to rise to greatest size in oven.
   e. Loaves flat on top may result from inadequate kneading.

9. COARSE GRAIN
   a. Too high temperature during rising.
   b. Rising too long or proofing too long.
   c. Oven too cool at first.
   d. Pan too large for size of loaf.
   e. Too much liquid.

I. BREADS

Apple Icing Bread

1 loaf bread dough
6 c. **Applesauce**, slightly warm

$^1/_4$ c. unsweetened coconut, optional

Use **One Loaf Recipe for Children**. Roll dough out $^1/_2''$ thick in large, flat baking pan, lining pan including sides. Prick dough with fork and pour on the warm **Applesauce**. Sprinkle with the coconut. Cover with flat pan or kneading board. Let rise until dough is double in thickness. Bake $1^1/_4$ hours at 350°. Leave in pan for one or more days. Heat before serving. Slice as a **Pie**.

One Loaf Recipe for Children

1 c. warm water
1 T. Karo **or** honey
1 T. yeast

1 t. salt
$2^1/_2$ c. whole wheat flour

Mix first three ingredients and let stand 10 to 15 minutes. Add remaining ingredients and squeeze between fingers, hand over hand until all is mixed and dough begins to turn loose from fingers. May need to add more flour. Turn onto floured board and knead well. Shape immediately into loaf, or let rise once or twice. Bake at 350° for 45 to 50 minutes.

Whole Wheat Bread

3 c. water
3 T. honey
3 t. salt

3 T. yeast
8 c. whole wheat flour, warmed in oven for 3–5 minutes, at 275°

Have all ingredients warm and work in a warm room. Mix the first three ingredients in a blender or bowl. Add yeast and flour to the mixture in a large mixing bowl. Work together well by squeezing through fingers. Do this step well and kneading will be unnecessary. Add flour if needed. Keep the dough sticky as too much flour added makes a flat loaf. As soon as the dough begins to turn loose from the fingers, flour the hands and the bowl to prevent sticking. Let rise in bowl, set in a warm place, covered, until double in bulk. Cut in 3 parts with a sharp knife and place in loaf pans or floured cans (large fruit juice cans are ideal). Shape loaves nicely, or pack down well in cans and allow to rise until double in bulk. Place in preheated 400° oven for 15 minutes. Reduce heat to 350° for about 30 minutes. Remove from pans and cool on wire rack or several thicknesses of towels so air can circulate around them. Allow to age for 1–3 days before eating. Variation: For **Raisin Bread**, add $1^1/_2$ cups raisins to the dough.

Bold Print indicates items listed in the INDEX

I. BREADS

Rye Bread

Use the same recipe as for **Whole Wheat Bread** except that the 8 cups of flour are of mixed grains. A good loaf to start with has about 4–5 cups of whole wheat flour, 1–3 cups of unbleached white flour and 1–2 cups of rye flour, the total to equal about 8 cups. Do not use more than 2 cups of rye flour as it has little gluten to trap air bubbles.

Oatmeal Buns

Use the recipe for **Whole Wheat Bread** but use 6 cups unbleached white flour and 3 cups rolled oats instead of the 8 cups of whole wheat flour. DO LITTLE KNEADING. Form into buns after one rising. Bake at 400° for 20 to 30 minutes. Cool. Do not serve until next day. Place in tightly closed casserole to warm before serving. Whole wheat flour may be used in this recipe. Less is required than of unbleached white flour to make a dough of good consistency.

Soy Bread

Use the **Rye Bread** recipe but substitute soy flour for rye flour. This recipe makes good rolls. To make **Parkerhouse** or **Cloverleaf rolls**, cut the ball of dough for each roll, after it has been placed in muffin tin, with a scissors by inserting one prong in center and cutting in three or four directions, turning scissors. After rising the centers are together and the tops fall apart. Bake at 400° for 20 to 30 minutes.

Bagels

2 c. warm water	2 c. whole wheat flour
3 T. yeast	3 t. salt
3 T. honey	3½ c. whole wheat flour

Mix the first four ingredients and allow it to double in bulk. At the same time mix the next two ingredients along with any kind of seed, nut, or dried fruit desired. **Bagels** are good plain but may be made with raisins, chopped, dried apples, or other small seed or chopped nut, onion flakes or chips, etc. Add to the original mixture. Knead well. Pinch off small portions about the size of a small tangerine. Roll into a rope about 5″ long and ½″ to ⅓″ in diameter. Shape this rope into a ring. Drop into vigorously boiling water: use 3 quarts, salted with 3 tablespoons salt if desired. Allow **Bagels** to remain in the water until they float to the top (about 3 minutes). Remove, drain, and place on floured pan. Bake at 425° for 30 minutes.

Bold Print indicates items listed in the INDEX

I. BREADS

Russian Rye Bread
Pumpernickel

Mix the following ingredients and let stand 10 minutes:

1 qt. water, warm enough to warm up molasses	1 T. salt
	1 pkg. yeast
1 c. dark molasses	

Then add the following ingredients slightly warmed in the oven. Let stand 15 minutes.

3 c. rye flour	6 c. whole wheat flour

Knead, adding 2–4 cups unbleached white flour to make smooth and elastic dough. Allow a rising period as in **Whole Wheat Bread**. Make small loaves. Bake 1 hour at 350°.

Swedish Almond Braid

2 T. yeast	$^1/_2$ c. wheat germ **or** wheat bran
$^1/_2$ c. warm water	1 t. salt
$2^1/_2$ c. whole wheat flour	$^3/_4$ c. honey
$2^1/_2$ c. unbleached white flour	$^1/_2$ t. ground coriander
$^1/_4$ c. slivered almonds, optional	$1^1/_2$ c. hot water

Sprinkle yeast on warm water, stir and let stand 10 minutes. Pour hot water in bowl, and add honey, salt, coriander and wheat germ. Beat in unbleached white flour and enough whole wheat flour to make a stiff batter. Beat well, then add yeast mixture and beat again. Add enough additional whole wheat flour to make a stiff batter. Cover and let stand in warm place until double in bulk (about an hour).

Turn out on floured board and knead until smooth. Divide dough into two portions. Divide one portion into three equal pieces. Roll each piece into a rope 12″ to 14″ long. Braid the ropes together on a floured cookie sheet, and let rise until almost double in bulk. Brush with warm **Soy Milk** and cover with slivered almonds (optional). The other half of dough can be made into another braid. One may be frozen for another day. Bake in preheated oven at 350° for 30 to 40 minutes or until nicely brown.

Doughnuts

Use recipe and directions for **Swedish Almond Braid** except that dough is placed on floured counter top rolled out to $^1/_3$″ thick. Cut with a doughnut cutter. Place on floured cookie tin to rise. Bake at 375° 15 to 20 minutes. Use a glaze of **Carob Sauce** if desired immediately before serving. Makes 36 doughnuts.

Bold Print indicates items listed in the INDEX

I. BREADS

One Hour Whole Wheat Bread
4 small loaves

YEAST MIXTURE:
>   1 c. warm water
>   3 pkg. yeast **or** 3 T. dry yeast
>   1 T. honey **or** molasses
>   Mix and let stand 10 minutes.

SPONGE MIXTURE:
>   3 c. hot water, from tap
> $1/_3$ c. honey
> $1^1/_2$ c. flour
>   Mix and let stand while yeast is getting ready to be mixed in.

ADD LATER:
> $1^1/_2$ T. salt
>   Approximately $7^1/_2$ cups whole wheat flour or only enough to make soft
>   dough consistency.

Everything must be measured, warm, and ready to go. Warm the flour as whole wheat is often kept in the refrigerator to keep the germ from becoming rancid. Sponge must be lukewarm before yeast is added. When 10 minutes are up, add yeast mixture. Let stand 15 minutes. Add salt and flour. Must be a soft dough—not too stiff. Knead if desired up to 10 minutes, but may knead only until smooth. Put right into pans, whether bread, rolls, rings, etc. Loaves may be shaped round and placed in large, covered casseroles to prevent a dry skin from forming on the tops during the proofing period. Bake in the casserole after loaves have doubled in bulk. Place in a cold oven set at 250° for 15 minutes. If loaves are not high enough at that time, leave at that temperature for 5–10 minutes more. Turn oven to 350° and bake bread until done. Remove foil or casserole cover when oven is turned up.

For sweet rolls use hot pineapple or apple juice instead of hot water in sponge.

Roll out some dough to $1/_2$", spread with dates or date sauce (water and dates heated), roll up as a **Jelly Roll** and form into a **Horseshoe**. Score top layer in several places to expose some of the dates.

Make three long ropes to make a braid, using apples, almonds, or raisins down the center.

Make pretty **Napkin Rolls** by rolling triangles of dough starting the roll with one of the flat sides and ending with the point of the triangle. Sprinkle sesame seed on top.

Use about half of the dough to make 4 small pizza crusts. Roll or press into round or rectangular pizza pans. Bake about 25 minutes. Store 1–3 days before making pizzas.

Bold Print indicates items listed in the INDEX

I. BREADS

Whole Wheat Yeast Crackers

3 c. whole wheat flour, about
1 c. warm water
1 T. dry yeast

1 t. honey
1 t. salt

Add enough whole wheat flour (about 1$\frac{1}{2}$ cups) to make a soft batter. Let stand 10 to 15 minutes in a warm place. Then add more flour (about 1$\frac{1}{2}$ cups) to make a dough. Knead thoroughly. Divide into four portions and place each portion on a floured cookie sheet. Roll very thin with a floured dowel. Score into crackers. Let stand 30 minutes in a warm place. Bake at 250° about 1 hour until light brown. They are delicious!

Yeast Corn Bread

Let stand 5 minutes:

4$\frac{1}{2}$ c. warm water
$\frac{1}{4}$ c. honey

3 T. yeast

Mix in bowl:

3 c. corn meal
3 c. whole wheat flour
3 c. white flour **or** 2 c. whole wheat,
   1 c. quick oats

1 c. water
1 T. salt

Add yeast mixture, mix well. Place in oiled baking dish. Let rise 15–30 minutes. Bake at 350° for 45 minutes or until golden brown.

Diastatic Malt
(Use in sugar-free breads)

1 c. wheat berries

Put the whole grains of wheat into a wide-mouth glass jar and cover with nylon net, cheesecloth, or a clean mesh dishcloth or wire screen. Secure with a jar ring or rubber band. Cover with lukewarm water overnight. Rinse daily or twice daily for about two days. When the little sprouts are about the same length as the grains pour the sprouts out onto two large baking sheets. Dry in the oven at no higher temperature than 150°, about 8 hours. When thoroughly dry, grind to a fine flour in blender or mill. Use one teaspoon in a loaf of bread instead of one tablespoon of honey. Keeps in the refrigerator tightly closed for months.

Bold Print indicates items listed in the INDEX

Corn Muffins
Use also as **Corn Bread**

2 c. **Soaked Soybeans**   2 t. salt
2 c. water $1/4$ c. raw oats
2 T. honey, optional   2 c. corn meal

Place the first five ingredients in the blender and whirl until smooth. Pour into the corn meal. Mix well. Fill floured muffin cups. Bake in preheated oven at 400° for 35 to 40 minutes. Serve warm, rewarmed, or cold. Use for breakfast with oatmeal and **Apple-sauce**, or for a dinner bread. Does well as a loaf. Bake $1-1^1/_2$ hours for loaves.

NOTE: There is an enzyme in many soybeans which is released on crushing the bean. It is this enzyme that imparts a "beany" flavor, but the flavor develops only if the enzyme is allowed to work on the pulp after crushing the bean. Heat destroys the enzyme. Therefore it is well to preheat the oven, and work rapidly to prevent prolonged action of the enzyme after blending the beans.

Barley Cakes

$1^2/_3$ c. barley flour $1/2$ c. **Soaked Soybeans**
$1/2$ t. salt $1^1/_2$ c. water

Put all ingredients, except flour in blender and grind fine. Pour into bowl and add flour. Beat for about 1 minute. Dip with a large spoon onto floured pans, and bake at 375° to a nice brown, approximately 20–30 minutes.

Wheat Gems

2 c. whole wheat flour $1/4$ t. salt, optional
$1^1/_3$ c. water, about

Make a stiff dough using more or less water depending on the moisture content of the flour. Pinch off portions of dough about the size of a walnut and roll into a smooth, round ball. Place directly on the ungreased oven rack. Bake at 350° about 20 to 40 minutes until very lightly brown. Gems will turn loose from the oven rack when brown enough. These are chewy and delicious.

Bold Print indicates items listed in the INDEX

I. BREADS

Aerated Oatmeal Gems

1^1/$_3$ c. water
^{1}/$_2$ t. salt
pinch of herbs, optional

1 t. honey, optional
1^1/$_3$ c. rolled oats
^{1}/$_2$ c. whole wheat flour

Mix all ingredients to a smooth batter, and set in a very cold place overnight. Beat a few hard strokes with a spoon, and dip while still cold into hot floured iron gem pans, and bake in preheated oven at 350° to a nice brown, about 1 hour.

NOTE: Only iron gem pans should be used for aerated breads, as it is largely the contrast between the hot irons and the cold batter which causes the expansion of the gems.

Popovers

2 c. whole grain flour
^{1}/$_4$ c. sesame seed

1^1/$_2$ c. water
^{1}/$_2$ t. salt

Mix ingredients in blender until seeds are ground. Heat floured pan in oven at 425°. Quickly pour **Popovers**, using about 2–3 tablespoons of batter on the hot pan for each. Place in oven for 6–8 minutes. Then reduce heat to 375° for about 8 minutes until edges are browning. Toast 1–2 minutes under broiler to give a light brown color. Watch carefully.

Corn Gems

2^1/$_2$ c. corn meal
2 t. salt
2^1/$_2$ c. cold water

^{1}/$_2$ c. whole wheat flour
2 T. Karo
6 T. heaping, **Soaked Soybeans**

Mix flours. Whiz all other ingredients. Combine and heap into floured corn dodger irons, preheated. Bake at 375° for 45 minutes. Serve hot. Yield: 7 gems.

Spoon Bread

2 c. hot water
1 t. salt

1 c. sifted corn meal

Blend and boil the above ingredients until thick. Add 2 cups cooked, canned, or raw whole kernel corn. Whiz until creamy. Should the mixture be too thick for the blender to handle, add a little water. Pour into flat floured baking pan or casserole. Bake at 400° for 1^1/$_2$ hours or until golden brown. Keep the casserole covered until shortly before **Spoon Bread** is done. Serve hot or cold.

Bold Print indicates items listed in the INDEX

I. BREADS

Boston Brown Bread

4 c. whole grain flours
$1/_3$ c. molasses
1 c. raisins
2 c. water

$1/_2$ c. sunflower seed **or** nuts
1 T. grated orange rind
1 t. salt

Use corn meal, rye, barley, buckwheat, or whole wheat flours, any two or only one. Mix all ingredients and pour into a floured pyrex or steel mixing bowl. Set inside a covered kettle which contains about 1–2 cups of boiling water. Steam for 2 hours. (See diagram below.) Cool and slice thinly. Delicious when spread with **Applesauce** as a main dish at breakfast. Variation: This bread may be used for a vegetable meal by substituting 1 cup cubed or shredded sweet potato raw or baked, for the raisins. A coarser texture may be obtained by using $3^1/_2$ cups of flours and 1 cup of wheat bran. Add with this another full cup of water.

Covered Steamer

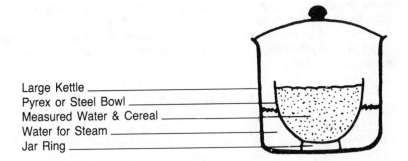

Large Kettle
Pyrex or Steel Bowl
Measured Water & Cereal
Water for Steam
Jar Ring

Date-Bran Muffins

3 c. shredded apples
$2^1/_4$ c. bran
$1/_2$ c. water
$2^1/_4$ c. oats

$1^1/_2$ t. salt
8–9 dates, chopped
6 T. nuts, chopped

Grind oats dry in the blender to make coarse flour. Mix all ingredients and let stand to wet oats and bran. Pack lightly into muffin pans. Heap into muffin shapes as they do not rise. Bake at 350° about 35 minutes. Yield: 12 muffins.

Variations: Use 1 cup chopped raisins instead of dates. To use for vegetable meals, leave out fruit and use $4^1/_2$ cups shredded sweet potato.

Bold Print indicates items listed in the INDEX

I. BREADS

Corn Fritters

$1^1/_2$ c. whole kernel corn
$^1/_3$ c. water
$^3/_4$ c. whole grain flour
$^1/_4$ t. salt

$^1/_4$ c. wheat germ **or** bran
2 T. soy flour
$^1/_4$ c. onions (or raisins for a fruit
    meal)

Lightly blend corn, onion or raisins, and water in blender. Add other ingredients. Drop by teaspoons onto floured cookie sheet. Bake at 350° for 8–10 minutes until brown on bottom. Bake for about 2 minutes under flame until tops are golden brown. Very good with raisins for a fruit meal.

Carrot Corn Bread or Apple Corn Bread

4 c. corn meal
1 c. **Soaked Soybeans**
1 T. salt
1 c. water

2 c. whole wheat flour
4 c. carrot pulp from juicer, **or** grated
    carrots

Grind **Soaked Soybeans**, salt, and water in blender until fine. Mix all ingredients. Add enough water to make the consistency of corn bread dough. More water will be needed for pulp from juicer. Pour into baking pan 1″ deep. Bake at 350° 1 hour or until golden brown. For a fruit meal substitute apple pulp or grated apples for carrots. May use grated sweet potato instead of carrots.

Gem Dandies

2 c. corn meal
2 c. whole grain flour, any kind
4 c. rolled oats

1 c. sesame seed, optional
$5^1/_2$ c. water
2 t. salt

Whirl the water, oats, salt, and sesame seed in the blender until most of the seed are chopped but part are still whole. Pour into the flour and meal. Mix well. Dip by large spoonsful onto a floured cookie tin. Bake at 350° for about 1 hour, or until lightly browned. Delicious gems! Variation: whirl 1–2 bananas in place of 1–2 cups of the water in the recipe for a delicious bread for a fruit meal.

Sweet Potato Muffins

1 c. finely shredded sweet potatoes
$1^1/_4$ c. rolled oats
$^1/_3$ c. wheat germ **or** bran
$^1/_2$ c. water

$^1/_2$ t. salt
$^1/_4$ c. unsweetened coconut,
    optional

Blend half of the oats to flour or use all quick oats. Mix the water and salt. Mix the shredded potatoes, coconut, and all the oats. Pour the wet ingredients into the potato-oat mixture. Stir well. Shape into small muffins, heaped up on top. Bake at 350° for 25 to 45 minutes, until golden brown.

I. BREADS

Simple Corn Muffins

$^1/_4$ c. shredded coconut, optional
$1^1/_2$ c. corn meal
$^1/_4$ c. whole wheat flour

$1^1/_3$ c. water
1 t. salt, scant

Mix all ingredients. Let stand 20 to 30 minutes before shaping muffins. Bake 45 minutes at 350°. Yield: 6 small muffins. May be baked in pan and cut in squares for serving.

Corn Pones

3 c. corn meal
4 T. ground unroasted peanuts, optional

1 c. boiling water
1 t. salt

Combine all ingredients and stir 2–3 minutes. Add more water if needed to make stiff dough. Cool. Put onto floured baking sheet by $^1/_4$ cupfuls. Flatten slightly with fork. Bake 40 minutes at 325°. Serve with **Fruit Sauce** for breakfast, or with gravy for dinner.

Hush Puppies

1 c. grits, stoneground best
1 c. onions, chopped

3–4 c. water
1 t. salt

Bring water to boil, add grits and salt. Cook for 1 hour. Cool until grits begin to get slightly stiff. Important not to overcool. Add onions. Spoon onto floured baking sheet. Cool to congeal fully if not already stiff. Bake at 425° for about 30 to 60 minutes. Give 1 minute under broiler if necessary to get slightly browned.

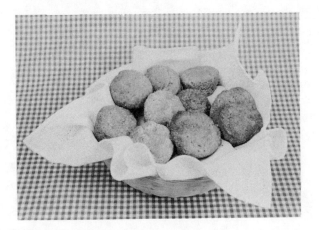

Bold Print indicates items listed in the INDEX

I. BREADS

Baked Corn Crisp

1 qt. whole kernel corn   1 t. salt

Add only enough water to cream in your blender. Pour $\frac{1}{2}$" thick in pan, or make flat patties, using 1 tablespoon for each patty. Bake at 375° for 1–2 hours until quite brown around the edges. Patties require only about 30 minutes.

Corn Fritos

2 c. fine corn meal   4 c. boiling water
1 t. salt

Mix salt and water and pour into the corn meal while stirring in a large mixing bowl. Use enough water to make thin enough to pour. Spread $\frac{1}{4}$" on floured baking pans. Sprinkle if you wish with food yeast, sesame seed. Bake at 250° until completely dry and crisp (1–2 hours).

Tortillas

2 c. fine corn meal $\frac{1}{2}$ t. salt
1 c. water

Mix and make into about 6 balls the size of a small apple. Roll each ball very thick with a dowel or rolling pin between sheets of waxed paper. Bake slowly on burner in hot, ungreased, heavy iron skillet, turning to brown both sides.

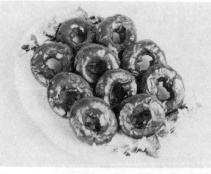

Doughnuts (See pages 16 and 18)

Bold Print indicates items listed in the INDEX

I. BREADS

BREAD IN THE DIET

Milk should not be used in the place of water when making bread. Its use is an additional expense and actually makes yeast bread less wholesome. The milk tends to encourage improper fermentation in the bread, developing substances that are harmful to the health, as described in the discussion of cheese. Bread dough and the fully baked bread should not be allowed to sour. The so-called sour-dough bread is unwholesome. Many times sprouted wheat bread dough is allowed to sour during the preparation phase. There is often a faint taint of sourness in the finished product. Even when there is no noticeable sour taste, there may be products of fermentation in the bread if the dough has been improperly handled. Good yeast bread will be light and sweet. Unleavened breads will be sweet. They may be chewy but should not be unpleasantly so, to endanger the dental structures or cause injury to the lining of the mouth. Individuals vary greatly in what they consider a pleasant consistency. Some will call a quick bread item a "delightful treat" that another calls "sad bread." In quick breads, a certain toughness or hardness may be very enjoyable if the shape of the bread is such that it can be easily handled.

Carefulness and much thought are required to make good bread. A good cook of a former era, Ellen White, has said that the making of good bread is a religious duty for every girl and woman, and that soda and baking powder and "such compounds" should not be used to compensate for a lack of caretaking by the cook. Saleratus in any form should not be taken into the stomach. It is likely that there is no baking soda or baking powder on the market that will not damage either the food it is used in, or the person who uses it. The quick breads (using no leavening agents) or yeast raised breads represent the healthful breads. With persistence and care every cook can become really proficient in the making of bread. Since bread is the real staff of life, every girl and woman should work at it until she becomes an excellent baker.

HIGH PROTEIN DIET

It is usually assumed that a high protein diet is entirely harmless. That this is not true is well attested by both animal experimentation and population studies. Reports in prominent medical journals of the dangers of high protein feedings have been largely overlooked until very recent times. Animals have their lives shortened considerably by a diet containing liberal quantities of protein. Diets containing about 10% of the calories in the form of protein seem to be the best in regard to status of health and length of life. As the amount of protein increases, growth is faster **and** life is shorter. Further, the kidneys may enlarge up to 50% bigger than in animals on a "normal" or "low" protein diet. Most animals get kidney disease while on prolonged high protein intake; many also get cancers. It is definite that the human body is overworked in converting protein into energy, and the process may not be without danger. It is also a process which is expensive, since the cost of protein foods generally runs much higher than complex carbohydrate foods. Athletes show greater energy and endurance on high carbohydrate diets. In every way it seems proper to take the most of our food in the form of carbohydrates. About 75% of calories as complex carbohydrates appears to promote the best functioning of all parts.

I. BREADS

DIGESTION

The digestion of food is a most difficult process. It is the changing of energy stored in foods to a form that the energy can be used as needed in making heat or doing work. Digestion ideally begins in the mouth. If the mouth phase is bypassed or half done, the work of digestion cannot be fully accomplished. Small bites should be taken and the food thoroughly chewed. The food should turn to a cream by the mastication process before it is swallowed. The more concentrated the food the more necessary it is to chew thoroughly and mix with saliva.

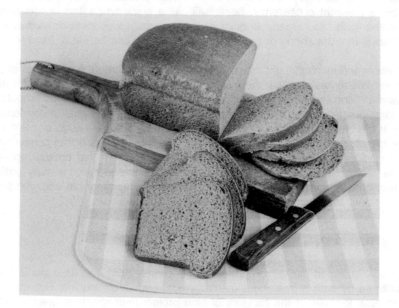

Whole Wheat Bread, page 14

Bold Print indicates items listed in the INDEX

I. BREADS

WEIGHT LOSS

When beginning a program of reducing the number of meals taken to two, or at most three; or when reducing the fats used in cooking or serving, many individuals will experience a weight loss, especially if there are factors such as anxiety, other changes in lifestyle, an increase in exercise, etc., that occur at the same time as the dietary changes. A modest weight loss is to be expected, and is usually not undesirable. Unless one loses strength or begins to feel bad, to lose weight is not a sign that there is a disease process going on. To maintain body weight 5–10% below the average weight for Americans seems desirable. Length of life, level of productivity, and sense of well-being all seem to be better if one is less than average weight by a few pounds. Remember that the lowering of the calories from the diet in the form of fat may represent 300 to 1000 calories each day. If these calories are not replaced by additional calories in the form of complex carbohydrates, weight loss can be considerable. In fact, for those who are overweight, the adoption of a fat free diet is usually the most effective, painless, and nutritionally sound method of weight loss.

For those who are thin at the beginning of a fat free diet, menus which will provide between 1500 and 2200 calories daily for sedentary workers should be provided. The complex carbohydrates are handled better by the body than any other nutrient, **even** if one has diabetes!

OVERNOURISHMENT MORE DANGEROUS THAN UNDERNOURISHMENT

By far a more dangerous possibility in this country is that of overnutrition rather than undernutrition. If one is using whole grains, a wide variety of fruits and vegetables, and avoiding "empty calories," there is little chance of a healthy person's becoming undernourished. On the other hand, our country is filled with people who are sick or disabled from the excess of nutrients they are taking. The excess is almost always in the direction of specific nutrient excesses, such as too much fat or refined carbohydrates. Degenerative diseases follow these specific excesses. It is now possible to predict which types of diseases a population will suffer from by studying the pattern of its nutritive excesses and deficiencies. Excesses in fats lead to heart and artery disease, malignancies, hepatic and digestive diseases. Excesses in refined carbohydrates lead to metabolic diseases such as diabetes, the "hypoglycemic syndrome" and stress-related diseases, liver and pancreatic disorders, neurologic and psychiatric conditions.

Bold Print indicates items listed in the INDEX

I. BREADS

Dumplings

$^1/_2$ c. water
$^1/_2$ t. salt

$^2/_3$ c. whole grain flour

Place the first two ingredients in a small saucepan and bring to a boil. Add flour. Stir until flour is absorbed and paste gathers into a ball. Cool until starch congeals and the dough "sets." Drop by teaspoons into any **Stew** such as **Beans**, **Potatoes**, **Tomatoes**, **Garbanzos**, etc. Simmer 10 minutes.

Yeast Dumplings

2 c. whole grain flour
2 t. onion salt
$^1/_2$ t. salt

2 t. yeast
$^3/_4$ c. water

Mix ingredients. Roll to $^1/_4$″ thickness on floured board. Cut into $^1/_2$″ squares with a sharp knife. Drop these squares into any lukewarm **Stew**, broth, **Garbanzos**, or other beans. Use plenty of liquid (about 8 cups) as dumplings will thicken the liquid. Allow to rise while lukewarm until they float. Quickly bring to a vigorous boil. Then gently simmer 1 hour. Refrigerate in same pot. Serve reheated next day, as yeast products should not be eaten on same day the yeast grows.

Lasagne Noodles

$1^1/_4$ c. whole wheat flour
1 c. unbleached white flour

1 c. warm water

Mix all ingredients well, and roll out on a floured board to $^1/_8$″ thickness. Sprinkle with flour, top and bottom. Roll extra flour in. Cut into $1^1/_2$″ strips. Dry in air or 200° oven until all trace of moisture is gone. Store in paper bag in cupboard.

Soy Noodles

$^1/_2$ c. **Soy Base**
1 t. salt

$1^1/_2$ c. whole wheat **or** unbleached white flour

Make a stiff dough. Add water if needed. Roll out as thin as possible on heavily floured board. Dry 1 hour. Cut into thin strips. Place in sun or 200° oven until entirely dry. Store in a dry place or in refrigerator until needed.

Bold Print indicates items listed in the INDEX

Macaroni or Spaghetti

$2^1/_3$ c. whole wheat flour   1 c. warm water
$^1/_4$ c. soy flour

Mix all ingredients into a ball. Roll out on a heavily floured board to $^1/_8$" thickness. Sprinkle with flour and roll the added flour into the dough. Allow to dry for about half an hour. Cut into $^1/_2$" strips for macaroni and $^1/_4$" strips for spaghetti. Dry thoroughly in sun or in 200° oven. Store in a paper bag in cupboard.

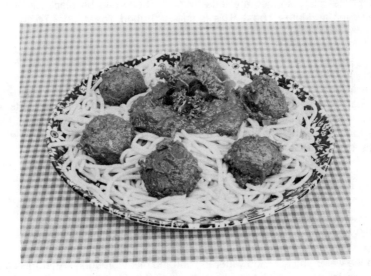

Spaghetti and Burger Balls, page 94

Bold Print indicates items listed in the INDEX

I. BREADS

Breading Meal

1 c. fine bread crumbs, made in blender   1/2 t. salt
1/2 c. yeast flakes   1 T. onion salt

Dry crumbs in oven until all traces of moisture are gone. Mix ingredients. Store in a dry place up to 1 year.

Zwieback
Melba Toast

Twice baked bread is very digestible. Make some **Melba Toast** from each batch of bread. Cut very thin slices and place directly on the oven rack. Bake at 175° to 225° until entirely dry and lightly browned. Another way is to pull chunks of bread off of a loaf in nice sizes for handling. Interesting shapes are thus formed. These can be placed in a pan to be dried in the oven as **Melba Toast**. This is called "**Pulled Toast**," or "**Toast Chunks**."

Croutons

Cut bread into about 1/2" to 3/4" squares. Place in pan in oven at 200° until entirely dry and lightly toasted. May be used in salads or soups or as a topping for desserts or roasts. Serve with cooked cereal to give a crusty morsel to chew with the soft cereal. Make very small **Croutons** and serve on steamed vegetables such as **Cauliflower**, new potatoes, **Asparagus**, or **String Beans**.

Chapatis

2 c. whole grain flour   1 c. water
2 T. nuts or seeds, ground   1/2 t. salt

Add salt to the water and stir. Add water to flour and mix thoroughly. After mixing it should be stiff like pastry dough. Add more flour if needed. If time permits, let it "rest" for half an hour. Make dough into balls about the size of a small egg. Roll each round or square about 6" in diameter. Bake **Chapatis** about 1 1/2 hours in 250° oven, or over burner in heavy skillet, until brown.

Bold Print indicates items listed in the INDEX

II. BREAKFASTS

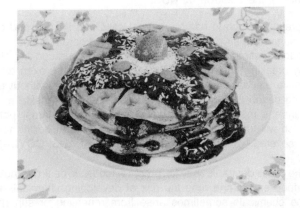

II. BREAKFASTS

For ideas and sample menus to make breakfast interesting and nutritious, turn to the section in the back of the book on MENUS.

Ground, whole grains are rich in natural mineral salts and flavors, and consequently require no oil and sugar in their preparation as do refined cereal grains, provided they are cooked long enough to eliminate any trace of raw flavor. Long cooking also improves the nutritive value by breaking chemical bondages which are not broken by shorter cooking nor by the digestive processes. A simple way to cook cereals without burning during a long, slow cooking period is to set a small saucepan or pyrex inside a large kettle. The small pan contains the measured grain, water, and salt. The larger pot contains some boiling water which will furnish the heat to keep the cereal at boiling temperature. Only the larger pot is covered. (See diagram on page 21, BREADS, **COVERED STEAMER**.)

Frying food is the least desirable way to prepare foods. It destroys nutrients, adds too much oil to the food eaten, and runs the risk of developing chemicals that are cancer-producing. These chemicals sometimes arise from reheating or superheating oils, especially in deep-fat frying.

MOST IMPORTANT MEAL

Breakfast should be a well planned, attractively served meal which contains about one half of the day's food requirements. Plenty of time should be allowed for eating. Breakfast is the most important meal of the day. The benefit to be derived from the food depends a great deal on how long the food spends in the mouth. Thorough chewing and an unhurried attitude are essential parts of this meal. No sense of haste should be allowed. Carefully avoid using too much concentrated foods, and over enriching foods with nuts, wheat germ, seeds, or salt and sugars. Rich foods are difficult for the body to handle. "Extra protein" is not needed. Eat a balanced diet according to the **Meal Planner** found in the MENU section of this book. Do not feel that your food is hurting you or is deficient. It is better to use whole fruit such as grapefruit and oranges rather than their juices. The pulp is valuable nutritionally, too. If you must buy canned fruit you can get it without sugar in most markets.

CEREALS

Many grains may be used cracked or ground coarsely. Try combining two different grains such as rice and buckwheat. Use as wide a variety as is possible, but do not mix more then two or three grains in one dish. Some of the less common grains are: Red whole wheat, rye (both rolled and whole grain), oat groats, **Brown Rice**, **Buckwheat Groats**, hulled barley, hulled **Millet**, and milo maize. Whole kernel cereals should be cooked for several hours. General directions are: 1 cup cereal, 1 teaspoon salt, and 3–4 cups water. They may be cooked in the following ways:

1. Slow baking dry, as first part of the cooking process (**Dextrinizing**). This step improves the flavor and shortens boiling time.
2. Slow baking in oven after water is added.
3. Cooking on burner by boiling or steaming.
4. Overnight cooking in electric fryer or bean pot, or pot-in-pot arrangement. (See diagram in section I.)

II. BREAKFASTS

THE USE OF FLOUR

When "flour" is called for in a recipe that does not use yeast, any kind may be used. Since yeast breads require wheat for their raising quality, it will be well to use barley, rye, buckwheat or other flours to thicken cereal or gravies, etc., rather than wheat. In this way a larger variety of nutrients may be obtained which will increase the constitutional strength of the family.

DEXTRINIZING GRAINS

Dextrinization is the changing of carbohydrates from long chains as in starches to shorter chains as in dextrins. It can be done by heating starches, also by enzymatic digestion. Dextrins are nearer to being sugars, therefore taste sweeter than starch. That explains why **Melba Toast** (which has been **Dextrinized** by the extra step in baking) tastes sweeter than regular bread. Grains, either in the whole grain berry, or as flour or grits, can be **Dextrinized** by heating dry either in a skillet on the burner, or in a baking pan in the oven. In the first instance, stir constantly on moderately high heat for 3 to 5 minutes. In the oven allow to bake dry at 325° for 5 to 10 minutes, watching carefully that it does not burn.

Bold Print indicates items listed in the INDEX

II. BREAKFASTS

Corn Meal Mush

1 c. corn meal	$^3/_4$ c. cold water
2$^1/_2$ c. boiling water	$^1/_2$ t. salt

Blend the corn meal with the cold water, add to the boiling water, and stir until it boils. Let boil quite rapidly until it begins to thicken. Reduce heat to low and let simmer for 20–40 minutes. Serve topped with **Applesauce**. Serves 3–4.

Millet
Use leftover as **Baked Millet**

1 c. millet	$^1/_4$ c. sesame meal (optional)
4 c. water	1 t. salt

Cook slowly 2 hours. Serve with **Fruit Sauce** as porridge. Serves 2–3. If any is left over, place in a refrigerator storage container until cold and congealed. Slice in $^1/_3$″ to $^1/_2$″ slices and bake at 350° for 45 to 60 minutes. Serve with **Fruit Sauce** or **Nut Cream**. Since baked millet may be held in the hand to be eaten, it can be used as bread with a spread. The slices may be rolled in wheat germ, bran, or crumbs before baking for crispy outside.

Buckwheat-Rice Cereal

$^1/_2$ c. buckwheat groats	5 c. water
1 c. brown rice	1 t. salt

Mix. Boil together for 1$^1/_2$ hours. Buckwheat has a strong flavor and is usually enjoyed better when mixed with a bland grain such as rice or millet.

Hominy Grits
"Grits" and "Baked Grits"

1 c. grits, stoneground, best	3–4 c. water
1 t. salt	

Bring water to boil, add grits and salt. Reduce heat and cook gently for 1–3 hours, the longer the better. Add more grits if they are still soupy after 10 minutes of cooking, as grits should never be served runny, but should pile up on a plate or in a bowl as soft mashed potatoes. While boiling, the steam should barely be able to bubble through the thick porridge. Serves 4. Always prepare a double recipe and store the extra in molds in the refrigerator. It congeals on cooling. Slice $^1/_2$″ thick. Bake for 1 hour at 350°. Serve **Grits** with **Wheatonnaise**, **Queen Fruit Sauce**, **Tomato Gravy**, or **Sautéed Breakfast Apples**. Serve **Baked Grits** with **Cereal**, **Waffle**, or **Dessert Toppings**. Make **Hush Puppies** for dinner from still-hot leftover **Grits**.

Rice Cereal—Risengrod

1 c. brown rice
4 c. water

1 t. salt

Cook over very low heat for two or more hours or all night on "warm" on electric stove. There may be a little water left by morning and the rice is almost creamy. Cook cereal 2 minutes while stirring to make creamy. Serve hot with a rich **Nut Cream** or **Wheatonnaise**. Serves 4.

Swedish Farina

$^2/_3$ c. rye flour
$2^3/_4$ c. water

1 t. salt
$^1/_2$ c. raisins

Whip the rye flour into the water. Add salt. Do not have any lumps in mixture. Stir rapidly while cooking over a high flame. When it starts to boil turn heat to low, add raisins, and cook for 10 minutes, stirring occasionally. The mush thickens while cooling. Serve with a **Nut Butter** lodged on side of bowl. Serves 2.

Bulgar Wheat
Rice, Rye, etc.

Roast whole kernel wheat or any whole kernel grain in oven at 350° for 15 to 20 minutes. Blend at high speed until it becomes a fine meal or coarse flour. All grains should be at least as small as millet. Store for use in recipes requiring **Bulgar** or **Cream of Wheat**.

Cream of Wheat

1 c. **Bulgar Wheat** (see recipe)
1 t. salt

$3^1/_2$ c. water

Sauté **Bulgar Wheat** in dry pan until nut-like fragrance appears. Cool slightly and add salt and water. Cook gently for 20 minutes or more. Serves 3–4.

Fruited Oats

4 c. boiling water
1 t. salt
$1^3/_4$ c. oats

$^1/_4$ c. dates or other dried fruit
1 large banana, chopped

Mix in the order given except for the banana, which is stirred in just before serving. Reduce the heat and let simmer for about 45 to 60 minutes. Serves 3–4.

II. BREAKFASTS

Lentil Porridge

1 c. lentils, raw
$^1/_2$ c. hulled millet
5 c. water

1 bay leaf
2 t. onion powder
salt, about 1$^1/_4$ t.

Bring to boil. Cook 1 hour. Remove bay leaf. Serve with melons for breakfast. Serves 4.

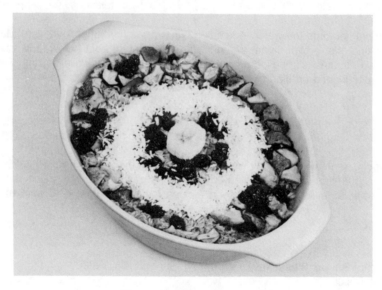

Fruited Oats, page 35

Bold Print indicates items listed in the INDEX

All Bran

1 lb. bran (8 cups)
1 c. water

1 c. molasses **or** Karo
(see sugarless type)

Mix water and molasses and pour into bran. Toss to moisten. Spread out in large, flat pans. Bake at 250° for 20 to 40 minutes, until dry, stirring occasionally. Use 1–2 table-spoons as a topping for any cereal porridge such as **Oatmeal**, **Corn Meal**, or **Swedish Rye**. For sugar-free diets, omit molasses and substitute 4 small apples, quartered, cored, and whirled in blender with water.

Maranola

8 c. rolled oats, ground to flour in blender
   or mill
$^1/_2$ to 1 c. water
1 c. finely ground coconut

2 c. cooked **Rice**, **Grits**, **Millet**,
   or other cereal
2 t. salt

Put all ingredients except oats in blender until smooth, using only enough water to blend. Pour ground oats and blended ingredients in a pan and mix. Place a sheet of hardware cloth over a shallow pan. Press the dough through the hardware cloth with a spatula. Bake 2–3 hours at 225°. This granola is so good, so nutritious, and so versatile, it is well worth the trouble to get a small piece of hardware cloth. Use **Maranola** as **Croutons**, **Dessert Topping**, on stews, as dry cereal, and as bread. Without oil it is quite hard. Cover for 10 minutes with **Fruit Sauce** to soften to an excellent chewing consistency.

Applesauce Granola

12 c. oats
3 apples, peeled, chopped small
3–4 c. applesauce

1 T. salt
1 T. vanilla

OPTIONAL INGREDIENTS: $^1/_4$ cup sweetening such as Karo or honey: 1 cup total of concentrated foods such as nuts, seeds, coconut, wheat germ (use no more than 1 cup total to keep the proportion down to 1:10 of these rich articles): carob or vanilla for fla-voring.

COOKING INSTRUCTIONS: Mix lightly all ingredients. Use little water. Spread out in pans and bake at 275° until entirely dry and lightly browned. Stir occasionally.

SERVING SUGGESTIONS: Place $^1/_2$ cup of **Granola** in a bowl and stir in $^1/_4$ cup **Ap-plesauce** or **Nut Milk**, **Stewed Fruit** or **Fruit Salad** make a good topping. **Carob Sauce** or any of the **Cereal**, **Waffle**, and **Dessert Toppings** listed in Section III are good **Gran-ola** toppings. Allow to set for about 10 minutes after sauce or **Nut Milk** is added. It will soften to a very good texture.

II. BREAKFASTS

Grapenuts
Low Calorie Cereal

Make **Granola** according to the recipe given. After thorough baking, grind in a seed mill or blender to a fine consistency. Serve as any dry cereal. Good mixed with **All Bran**, half and half.

Popcorn

$^1/_3$ c. popcorn, dipped in salty water

Place a large, covered kettle or fry pan on the stove at moderately high heat. Put the drained or dry popcorn in the pan. Shake the pan gently to keep the grains heating uniformly. Be prepared to pour up promptly as soon as popping ceases as the bottom kernels will burn. Serves 1–2. Save unpopped kernels to grind in blender and use in cooked cereals or roasts. Serve popcorn as a main dish at breakfast to be eaten dry with a sprinkle of salt, or with a **Fruit Sauce**, or **Nut Milk** poured over the kernels in a cereal bowl. **Popcorn** may be used instead of bread at dinner. **Popcorn** is a nourishing food; up to eighteen per cent of the calories are as protein!

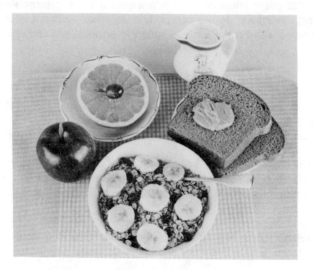

Granola, page 37

Bold Print indicates items listed in the INDEX

Corn Meal Squares
Cereal Fillets

$^1/_2$ c. corn meal
$^1/_2$ c. cold water
2 c. boiling water

1 t. salt
1 c. **Soy Base**, optional
Breading Meal

Mix the corn meal with the cold water. Pour into the boiling water and salt. Cook in the top of a double boiler until thick. Add the **Soy Base** and pour into a floured casserole or pan so the porridge is 1″ thick. Let it cool to congeal. Cut in 1″ squares. Roll in sesame seed, wheat germ, bran, bread crumbs, or **Breading Meal**, and bake at 350° until brown. **Rice**, **Grits**, **Millet**, **Oats**, or **Swedish Farina** may be used instead of the congealed **Corn Meal Mush** given in this recipe. Serve with a **Fruit Sauce** or maple syrup for breakfast, or use as a bread for either breakfast or dinner. A very versatile dish.

Rice Fritters

1 c. cooked rice, salted
$^1/_3$–$^1/_2$ c. flour

1 T. honey **or** Karo
2–4 T. water

Make a very stiff batter of the mixed ingredients. Form flat fritters or round balls. Roll in wheat germ. Bake at 350° for 45 to 60 minutes or to a golden brown. Serve with **Fruit Sauce**. Serves 2.

Oat Dodgers

3 c. oats
$^1/_3$ c. wheat germ
1 t. salt, scant

$^1/_3$ c. dates
1 c. water scant

Blend very lightly the last three items and combine with the dry. Press dough into small balls or ovals. Bake on ungreased tin at 300° for 1 hour. Serves 4–6 (20 balls 1$^1/_2$″).

Corn Dodgers

3 c. corn meal
$^1/_2$ c. unsweetened coconut, optional

2$^1/_8$ c. boiling water
1 t. salt

Mix and spoon onto floured cookie sheets. Bake at 375° for about 30 minutes. Makes 10 dodgers.

Bold Print indicates items listed in the INDEX

II. BREAKFASTS

Corn Meal Soufflé

2 c. boiling water	$3/4$ t. salt
$1/3$ c. corn meal	$1/4$ c. water
$1/4$ c. soy flour	

Pour the boiling water over the corn meal. Cook in the double boiler for 30 minutes, stirring occasionally. Mix $1/4$ cup water, salt, and flour, and add to the hot corn meal. Bake in baking dish about 1 hour at 350°. Serve with **Nut Cream** or **Coconut Gravy** as breakfast cereal or with **Seasoned Gravy** for main dish at dinner. Serves 2.

Baked Fruited Oats

Bring to a boil 2 cups water and 1 teaspoon salt. Add $1^1/2$ cups oats. Add 2 tablespoons sesame seed, or $1/2$ cup of raisins, or chopped dates, or other dried fruit. Put in floured casserole. Do not stir. Bake at 350° for 60 minutes. Serve with **Fruit Sauce** or juice. Variation: The items added after the oats may be left out for plain baked oatmeal. Serves 2–3.

Auf Lauf

Place a layer of leftover cereal or bread in the bottom of a baking dish. Next, spread a layer of dried or chopped fresh fruit, such as apple, over the cereal. Fill the baking dish with alternating layers of cereal and fruit. Top with chopped nuts or date nuggets. Pour **Nut Milk** or **Fruit Sauce** over layers until dish is half full. Bake at 350° for 45 minutes.

Apple Crisp

(See DESSERT section for this and many other fruit dishes that are low enough in concentrated sugars that they can be used readily as main dishes for breakfast.)

Musseli

1 c. quick oats	4 T. chopped nuts or
1 c. water, scant	sunflower seed
4 c. apples, grated or chopped	

Dextrinize oats lightly, about 10 minutes at 300°. Soak in water overnight. Just before serving add apples and nuts. Mix in some more water, juice, or **Soy** or **Nut Milk** as needed to adjust to proper consistency. Top with berries. Serves about 3.

Bold Print indicates items listed in the INDEX

Oat Waffles

8 c. rolled oats, lightly dextrinized in oven	1 T. salt
	8 c. water

Mix together and allow to stand overnight in refrigerator. Preheat waffle iron but do not allow to smoke. Use 1–1$\frac{1}{2}$ cups batter for each waffle. Bake each waffle 15 minutes before opening waffle iron. Place on bare oven rack at 175° to keep hot. Serve with hot strawberry sauce or any **Fruit Sauce**. Makes 5 waffles, 4 sections each. Try **Melba Toast Waffle**. Dry waffle entirely in oven at 200°. A dainty!

All Waffles

Soy Waffles, **Corn**, **Rye**, **Buckwheat**, or **Wheat Waffles** may be made by simply substituting part or all of the desired flour in the **Oat Waffles** recipe above. Keep the flours in the same proportion to water and salt.

Soy or Garbanzo Waffles

1 c. soaked garbanzos or soybeans	$\frac{1}{2}$ t. salt
1$\frac{1}{2}$ c. rolled oats	2$\frac{1}{4}$ c. hot water
2–4 T. nuts or seeds, optional	

Blend for $\frac{1}{2}$ minute. Bake 15 minutes in properly prepared moderate waffle iron using 1$\frac{1}{2}$ cups batter for each waffle. Yield: 2 waffles, 9″ each.

Pain Perdu
Leftover Bread Dish

MILK MIXTURE	BATTER
1 c. **Soy or Nut Milk**	$\frac{3}{4}$ c. whole grain flour
1 t. Karo	$\frac{1}{2}$ c. water
$\frac{1}{4}$ t. vanilla	1 T. Karo
pinch of salt	$\frac{1}{2}$ t. vanilla
	$\frac{1}{4}$ t. salt

Moisten 8 slices bread in the milk mixture and place slices on a floured baking pan. Mix the batter ingredients (try barley as the flour) and pour over the bread slices in the pan. Bake at 350° for about 30 minutes, or until lightly toasted. Serve with **Sesame Spread** or **Fruit Sauce**. Yield: 8 servings.

Bold Print indicates items listed in the INDEX

II. BREAKFASTS

French Toast

$\frac{1}{4}$ c. cashews **or** sesame seed
2$\frac{1}{4}$ c. water

$\frac{1}{2}$ t. salt
2 c. oat flour

Whirl the first three ingredients in blender. Pour into flour and stir. Dip about 12 slices of bread in this batter and bake at 400° for 10 minutes. Reduce heat to 350° until toast is nicely browned. Use broiler for last minute or two to develop brown on top if necessary. Yield: 12 servings.

Sesame Toast

Lightly toast bread under broiler on one side. Brush the other side with water and press wet side onto a plate of sesame seed. Now put untoasted, sesame side under broiler until toasted. Use care not to burn seed.

Garbanzo Toast

Liquefy or mash two cups of cooked **Garbanzos**. Add enough water or **Milk** to make the consistency of thick gravy. Heat in a heavy kettle or a double boiler. Season with salt to taste. Serve hot over **Melba Toast**, **Maranola**, or **Croutons**. Garnish with chopped parsley. Serves 4.

Corn Meal Pan-Cakes

1 c. whole grain flour
2 T. starch
$\frac{1}{3}$ c. corn meal

$\frac{1}{2}$ t. salt
1 c. water
3 T. soy flour

Put flour and meal in the oven at 350° for 5–6 minutes to lightly toast. Put all ingredients in blender and beat for 1 minute. Place by spoonsful onto floured pan. Bake about 15 minutes at 375° until golden brown. Turn broiler on for last 1–2 minutes to brown tops. May be used with **Fruit Sauce** as breakfast dish, or as **Chapatis** with vegetable stew, Indian style.

Corn Oat Waffles

3 c. water
2 c. rolled oats
1 c. corn meal

1 t. salt
1$\frac{1}{2}$ t. vanilla
$\frac{1}{4}$–$\frac{1}{2}$ c. sesame seed

Blend. Bake 12–15 minutes on moderate setting.

Bold Print indicates items listed in the INDEX

III. DAIRY PRODUCT SUBSTITUTES

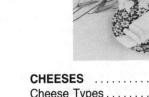

III. DAIRY PRODUCT SUBSTITUTES

INTRODUCTION

USES OF DAIRY PRODUCT SUBSTITUTES

The great increase in disease in cattle and the recognition of animal fat as a factor in the production of heart and artery disease have created a need for substitutes for dairy products which will be wholesome and appetizing. Most of these foods can be made at a fraction of the cost of the original article. Substitutes are generally easy to make and the flavors are so easy to alter that the cook can easily satisfy the particular tastes of her own family.

Nutritionally, many foods supply the elements of milk. Such common foods as greens, legumes (beans and peas), and whole grains will furnish an abundance of calcium and riboflavin, the two nutrients most likely to be missed when milk is omitted from the diet. There are, however, other qualities of dairy products that do not pertain directly to nutritional makeup of dairy products that must be supplied by suitable substitutes. A sauce to pour over cereals, an emulsion to use as a cream over vegetables and fruits, a butter to spread on bread, and cheeses that can be used not only as a dip but as melted or sliced foods. All these are suggested in this section.

FOOD YEAST AND GOUT

Use of both baker's and brewer's yeast should be made with caution. These food items are capable of raising the uric acid level of the blood. Elevated uric acid is associated with a serious metabolic disorder called gout. This disease is characterized by painful and swollen joints as well as other tissues. It is a form of arthritis. Small elevations in uric acid are not uncommon in our population. We should recognize, therefore, that people who are susceptible to developing gout are also not uncommon. All diabetics and their first degree relatives should be placed in this category. Foods that are high in purines cause the uric acid level to rise in the blood. Below is a list of high purine foods.

Meat and meat extracts	Mackerel and other fish	Goose and other poultry
Organ meats	Roe	Mincemeat
Shell fish	Sardines	Partridge
Anchovies	Gravy	Yeast, baker's and brewer's

All plant foods are low in purine content, but certain vegetables are higher than others, namely mushrooms, asparagus, spinach, and dry peas and beans.

Bold Print indicates items listed in the INDEX

Coconut Cream

2 c. water
$^1/_4$ c. unsweetened coconut
$^1/_4$ c. whole grain flour (barley best)

2 T. Karo **or** honey
$^1/_4$ t. salt

Liquefy water and coconut for 1 minute. Use unsweetened shredded or fresh coconut. Add remaining ingredients and mix. Stir until thickened over medium heat. Cover and simmer very gently for 10 minutes. Serve hot over cereals and desserts. Serve cold over fruit as a dressing.

Fresh Coconut Milk

1 c. fresh coconut
3 c. water including coconut liquid

1 t. honey
pinch of salt

Whiz until smooth in blender. May strain or use on cereal unstrained. Dried coconut may also be used.

Double Strength Soy Milk for Cream

Sort and soak $1^1/_3$ cups soybeans 2–3 hours or overnight. Drain. Let very hot tap water (140°) run slowly over beans in a pan about 5 minutes. Heat the blender by filling to the top with very hot water and let stand. Have kettle of boiling water ready. Drain beans, empty water out of blender and put in hot beans. Add $3^1/_2$ cups boiling water. Cover. Blend 3 minutes. Empty into a draining bag. Place in a large strainer. Squeeze (this is work!) until most of the liquid is extracted. Cook liquid in pre-heated double boiler 20 minutes. Chill. (This base has many uses: As a base for **Soy Milk** after diluting and flavoring with salt and honey; or as **Soy Yogurt** base.) When the beans are thus heated; the enzyme that gives a "beany" flavor by acting on the bean pulp, is quickly inactivated. This recipe has the most delicate flavor of the **Soy Milks**.

Sour Cream

2 c. **Nut Cream**
2 T. lemon juice

$^1/_8$ t. salt

Chill cream (use canned commercial soy milk if desired) and blend until foamy. Pour up. Add lemon juice and stir gently to thicken. Add salt or seasonings.

Bold Print indicates items listed in the INDEX

<u>MILK AND CREAM</u>

Banana Soy Milk

BASE

1 c. **Soaked Soybeans** $1^1/_2$ c. water

Blend 1 minute. Cook 1 hour in double boiler.

MILK

1 c. base $^1/_8$ t. salt
$3^1/_2$ c. water   1–4 bananas
1 t. vanilla

Blend well. Serve over cereal. Base stores 2 weeks. Variation: Omit bananas and add up to 1 cup leftover cereal and 1–3 tablespoons carob for a creamy, non-sweet cereal topping. Try also 2 cups strawberries with 2 tablespoons honey instead of the bananas.

Soy Base and Milk
With Flavor Variations

2 c. water   1 c. soy flour

Whirl in blender. Cook for 1–3 hours in double boiler. Store in refrigerator. To make **Soy Milk**, place 1 cup of **Soy Base** in blender. Add sufficient water to make the consistency of milk. Adjust the flavor of **Soy Milk** by any of the following suggestions. Add about $^1/_4$ teaspoon salt to each quart of milk made. Add a banana, if desired, to sweeten and flavor. The addition to the blender of $^1/_2$–1 orange, peeled and chopped, will cut the "beany" flavor which some species of soybeans have. Use also vanilla, almond extract, honey, lemon, or mint flavorings. Use a handful of nuts such as pecans to adjust the flavor. Whiz in an apple, or any other fresh or dried fruit, to give a fresh or sweet flavor. To thicken and make creamy, add up to 1 cup of any cooked cereal.

Carob-Peanut Butter Spread

2 bananas   2 T. carob
$^1/_2$ t. vanilla   2 T. honey

Blend smooth all of the ingredients. Add $^1/_2$ cup peanut butter and blend smooth.

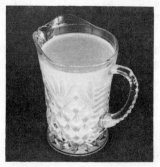

III. DAIRY PRODUCT SUBSTITUTES 47

MILK AND CREAM

Soy Sour Cream

1 c. **Soy Base**
1 T. Soyagen powder

¹/₄ t. salt
2 T. lemon juice

Thin **Soy Base** to consistency of cream. Mix first three ingredients in blender at high speed until creamy. Remove and add lemon juice. Use on potatoes as a sour cream substitute.

Sesame-Coconut Cream

2 c. boiling water
1 t. honey
¹/₄ t. salt
¹/₂ c. sesame seed

¹/₂ c. grated fresh coconut (dry, un-sweetened shredded may be used)

Liquefy and serve. May be strained if a smoother texture is desired. Dilute if necessary.

Vegetarian Cream

1 c. **Double Strength Soy Milk**
¹/₂ c. cooked **Millet**

¹/₂ t. salt

Blend for 1 minute and serve. This has many uses: As cream on vegetables, beans, grains, desserts, salads, or breads.

Nut Milk and Cream

	WATER	NUTS	SALT	FLAVORINGS
Milk	4 c.	1 c.	¹/₈–¹/₄ t.	Honey, vanilla, banana, or any fruit, carob, or maple flavoring.
Cream	2 c.	1 c.	¹/₈–¹/₄ t.	Same as above. Add leftover cereal to make more thick and creamy.
Butter	¹/₂–1 c.	1 c.	¹/₈–¹/₄ t.	Maple flavoring, onion, or garlic, paprika, or other yellow coloring.
Blend until as smooth as desired.				

Bold Print indicates items listed in the INDEX

III. DAIRY PRODUCT SUBSTITUTES

CEREAL, WAFFLE, AND DESSERT TOPPINGS, SPREADS

Fruit Sauce, Puddings, Custards

Fruit juices or fruit which has been canned, frozen, or dried may be made into delicious dishes for use over cereals and desserts by simply thickening them with flour, starch, tapioca, or agar. Use the following table for making the proper thickening, starting with 4 cups of fruit juice for the first 3 recipes, and 4 cups of stewed fruit with the stewing water for the last recipe.

	STARCH	FLOUR	TAPIOCA	AGAR	SWEETENER	SALT
Fruit Sauce	2–3 T.	4–6 T.	2 T.	2 T.	Varies with fruit	Pinch to 1 t.
Pudding	$1/3$ c.	$1/2$ c.	4 T.	4 T.	"	"
Custards	$1/2$ c.	1 c.	6 T.	4 T.	"	"
Hot, Stewed, Dry Fruit	1 T.	2–4 T.	"	2–4 T.	"	"

Mix gently while stirring. Serve hot or pour into molds and chill to thicken before serving.

Sesame Spread

$1/4$ c. sesame seed
1 T. Karo
2 apples

pinch of salt
2 T. **Soy Base**
1 small orange

Peel orange, remove seeds and place in blender. Quarter and core apple. Place all ingredients in blender and whirl to make a thick, soft butter consistency. Spread thickly on hot bread or toast and top with berries or **Fruit Sauce**; or use as milk substitute for cereal.

Fresh Applesauce

4–6 apples

1 orange

Chop each apple into several chunks for blender. Peel orange, chop, and remove seeds. Put orange in blender first to make liquid for blending. Blend together until smooth. May need to add a little water. Serve over cereal or bread for delicious breakfast treat.

Bold Print indicates items listed in the INDEX

Fruit Sauce

Place any available fruit or any combination of fruits, small or large proportions of leftover **Fruit Salad**, in blender with just enough water, milk, or fruit juice for the blender to whirl it. After fruit is well blended you may add small quantities of leftover cereal to make sauce more creamy. A sprinkle of salt often enhances the flavors and highlights the sweetness.

Raisin Sauce

Plump raisins by covering raisins with boiling water. Allow to stand overnight or boil for a few minutes until plump. Place in blender with additional water, if necessary, for blender to whirl it. Blend until smooth. If sauce is too watery may add leftover cereal, soy milk powder, nuts, or coconut to thicken.

Sauces to Use on Hot Cereal, Waffles, or Pancakes

There are numerous sweet sauces that make a dessert or cereal handsome and delicious. They are useful for the busy cook to make her meals a success. Whirl canned or frozen fruit of any kind in blender with liquid or other fruit juice or non-dairy milk.

A research report showed that of more than thirty fruits tested bananas are richest in vitamin B_6. It showed that bananas have 5.94 mg. of this vitamin per gram. The fruit next richest in vitamin B_6 is avocado at 4.5; then golden raisins at 3.33. Bananas are rich in magnesium. Magnesium and vitamin B_6 have been reported as favoring a normal level of cholesterol in the blood. Magnesium helps give steady nerves, a calm spirit, a strong digestive tract, and a keen mind. Small amounts of vitamins A, B_1, B_2, C, and the minerals calcium, phosphorus, and iron are found in bananas. They furnish small amounts of fat and protein. A banana of medium size, weighing $3^1/_2$ ounces, has 100 calories. Because bananas are quickly digested, they are a source of quick energy. A banana can be added to any of the sauces given in this section.

Fresh Apple Milk

Place 2 cups **Nut Milk** in blender. Add 3 or 4 washed apples which have been chopped into 1–2″ chunks. Stems must be removed, but seeds, cores, and skins will be chopped fine by most blenders. Blend 1–2 minutes.

Orange Sauce

May be handled as **Fresh Apple Milk**. Dry, juiceless oranges that would otherwise be discarded make good sauce by this method. The best way to make a delicious **Orange Sauce** is also the simplest: Peel the oranges, chop into quarters, place in blender, and grate fine. Seeds may be removed before blending if they are numerous. No fluid needs to be added as it makes its own juice.

III. DAIRY PRODUCT SUBSTITUTES

CEREAL, WAFFLE, AND DESSERT TOPPINGS, SPREADS

Sautéed Breakfast Apples

4 c. shredded apples with peelings   salt to taste
1 T. lemon juice

Heat shredded apples and lemon juice. Stir constantly for 3–4 minutes. Reduce heat, cover and continue cooking for 10 minutes. Serve with grits or over oatmeal as a topping. Serves 5–6.

Carob Sauce

1 c. water
2 t. vanilla
1–2 T. Karo **or** honey
$1/8$ t. salt

2–4 T. starch
2 T. carob powder
3 T. pecans, optional

Mix ingredients in blender, cook until starch is thickened. Make desired consistency by adding more or less starch. Serve over sweet **Rolls**, **Puddings**, **Doughnuts**, or as a spread for **Melba Toast**.

Fruit Juice Sauce

1 c. orange juice **or** any fruit juice   sprinkle of salt
1 T. flour

Mix and cook in saucepan until slightly thickened. Refrigerate. Serve on cereals or **Fruit Salads**. Serves 3–4.

Banana-Pineapple Sauce

2 small slices pineapple
2 c. water

1 medium sized banana
$1/8$ t. salt, scant

Combine in blender. More or less fruit may be added according to taste. Serves 3–4.

Tropical Cereal Sauce

1 c. pineapple juice $1/2$ banana

Liquefy in blender.

Bold Print indicates items listed in the INDEX

Queen Fruit Sauce

$2/3$ c. light-colored fruit juice **or**
    one large orange
2 T. lemon juice

1 T. Karo **or** honey
2 t. starch
$1/8$ t. salt

If orange is used, peel, remove seeds, and blend fine. Put all ingredients in a small saucepan and bring to a boil, stirring constantly. Do not boil, but allow to thicken.

NOTE: **Vegetarian Cream** or **Wheatonnaise** in the proportion of $1/3$ cream to $2/3$ sauce, added to the sauce when cold, is excellent.

Blackberry Sauce

2 c. blackberries, canned or fresh
$2/3$ c. water
1 T. lemon juice

1 T. starch
2 T. honey
sprinkle of salt

Blend ingredients and boil 4 minutes. If fresh berries are used add them last after boiling. Cool slightly before adding berries. Serve hot over breakfast cereal or toast. Good over hot puddings.

Cocopeanut Cream

1 c. water
$1/4$ c. coconut
3 T. Karo **or** 3 dates

$1/4$ c. peanuts, very lightly toasted
pinch of salt

Blend until smooth. Serve as cream substitute over cereals, fruit or desserts. Good over **Baked Sweet Potatoes** or **Butternut Squash**.

Banana Cereal Sauce

4 c. water
1 c. flour
2 bananas, chopped
1 t. vanilla

honey **or** Karo to taste
1 t. salt
$1^1/2$ c. frozen orange juice
    concentrate

Cook flour and water gently 20 minutes. Whirl in blender if not smooth. Pour into a serving bowl containing all the rest of the ingredients. Serve hot over cereal.

Vanilla Sauce

$1/4$ c. Karo
1 T. tapioca **or** 1 T. starch
$3/4$ c. water

1 slice lemon **or** orange with peel
1 t. vanilla flavor
$1/8$ t. salt

Mix the first four items. Boil for 5 minutes. Pour immediately into blender with salt and vanilla. Serve over cereals or stewed fruits. Keeps 2 weeks refrigerated.

Cheese Types

1. Cheeses which run, for sauces over vegetables (example, **Golden Sauce**).

2. Cheeses which spread or slice (example, **Nut Cheeses**).

3. Cheeses which melt (example, **Agar Cheese**) for use on **Pizza** and **Grilled Sandwiches**.

Chee Sauce

1 c. tomatoes **or** $^1/_2$ c. pimientos
1 c. water
$^1/_3$ c. lemon juice
$1^1/_2$ t. salt

1 t. onion powder, optional
$^1/_8$ t. garlic powder
2 T. sesame seed, optional
1 T. yeast flakes

Blend until smooth. Very good as a replacement for cheese in **Macaroni** or **Spaghetti** casseroles.

Golden Sauce

$^3/_4$ c. water
$^1/_2$ c. potatoes
$^1/_4$ c. carrots
1 T. food yeast

$^1/_2$ t. salt
1–3 T. lemon juice
1–2 T. nuts or seeds, optional

Liquefy ingredients in blender until smooth. Cook only if potatoes and carrots are raw, otherwise heat to serving temperature. This sauce is good on greens, grits or rice, vegetables and roasts. The flavor may be varied by whizzing in 1 cup tomatoes in place of carrots and water, and $^1/_2$ cup cooked cereals in place of potatoes. Use for grilled sandwiches by toasting open face under broiler.

Soy Cottage Cheese

1 c. soy grits
2 c. water

$^1/_2$ t. salt **or** onion salt

Stir ingredients together. Cook in double boiler without stirring 3–4 hours. Cool. Remove a portion and gently mix curds with enough lemon juice to make sour. Shape into a mound. Garnish with paprika and serve as cottage cheese. May be used instead of **Tofu** in the recipe for **Scrambled Tofu**. Make **Soy Grits** from raw or toasted soybeans, ground to grits in blender.

Bold Print indicates items listed in the INDEX

Scrambled Tofu
Soy Cheese

1/2 t. onion powder	1/2 t. paprika
1/2 t. vegetable salt, optional	2 c. cubed **Tofu or Soy Cottage**
1/2 t. salt, if needed	**Cheese**

Heat all ingredients in a skillet. Mix well with fork. Serve like scrambled eggs with toast. For variation: Add chopped green onions and garnish with parsley flakes.

Tofu
Oven Method

4 c. water	1/2 c. flour
2 1/4 c. soy flour	1/3 c. lemon juice
2/3 c. pimientos	1/4 t. garlic salt, optional
2 1/2 t. salt	1 T. food yeast

Place in blender and whirl until smooth. Pour into a small, floured loaf pan. Bake 2 hours at 275°. Keep in oven after turning off for another hour. Chill before turning out of pan. Peel off the brown skin on top and trim loaf to shape. Slice or cube for serving. Use on **Pizza**, on dinner platter, as **Scrambled Tofu**, in soups, salads, or sandwiches.

Tofu
Pressure Cooker Method

1 c. soy flour	juice of 2 lemons
3 c. boiling water	

Mix the flour with enough cold water to make a medium paste. Add to the boiling water and cook gently 5 minutes. Remove from heat. Add the lemon juice and stir only once. Do not disturb again until cool. Strain the curd through cheesecloth. Twist top of cheesecloth and set a weight on curd in a colander until all liquid is expressed (2–3 hours). Place curd in a stainless steel or pyrex bowl and pressure-cook for 30 minutes at 5 pounds, or in kettle for 1 hour. Use in sandwiches, **Scrambled Tofu**, or salads.

Tofu
Third Method

Soak 2 1/2 cups of dry soybeans overnight. Blend beans with water using 1 cup beans to 4 cups water until the beans are used up. Pour into colander lined with a thin linen towel, squeeze out liquid. Pour into large kettle as it boils over readily. Boil 3 minutes, then turn off heat. Add 1/2 cup of lemon juice or 1 tablespoon epsom salts, dissolved in 1/4 cup warm water. Wait 5–10 minutes until milk curdles well. Then gently lift the curd into a colander lined with a clean towel. Fold towel over curd and put a weight on top, such as a plate holding a 2 quart jar of water. Let drain well (2–3 hours).

CHEESES
_____

Agar Cheese

$1/4$–$1/2$ c. agar
$1^1/_2$ c. water
$3/_4$ c. sesame seed
1 can pimientos

1 t. salt
1 t. onion or garlic powder
2–8 T. lemon juice

Soak agar in water about 5 minutes and boil gently until clear. While agar is boiling, place next 5 ingredients in blender and whirl until smooth. Add hot agar and whirl $1/_2$ minute. Add the lemon juice last and mix for only a second. Pour immediately into mold and set in refrigerator to cool. Slice thinly onto a platter and garnish with parsley branches. Another beautiful way to serve this cheese is to cut into 1" cubes. Place in a black or white bowl. Variation: Try $1/_4$ cup food yeast or $3/_4$ cup cashews instead of sesame seed.

Nut Cheese

1 c. whole wheat flour
1 c. corn meal
$1^1/_2$ t. salt

$1^1/_2$ c. warm water
$3/_4$ c. **Nut Butter**
1 qt. canned tomatoes

Dextrinize flour and meal at 350° for 6–8 minutes. Mix water and **Nut Butter**. Blend all ingredients. Pour into round floured tins. One recipe fills three #2 cans. Set cans in casseroles and bake 1 hour at 350° with covers on, removing during last 15 minutes to brown tops. Delicious sliced hot or cold. Variation: try $1/_2$ cup chopped olives, celery, or onion. Salt, food yeast, sage, or pimiento may be added for color and flavor.

Soy Yogurt

1 qt. **Soy Milk**, regular strength
1 t. **Yogurt** from previous batch (or culture purchased commercially)

Sterilize **Soy Milk** by boiling. Cool to lukewarm. Add the culture material and stir well. Incubate at 98° for 8 hours or until junket consistency appears. Chill without stirring. This procedure does not putrefy the soybeans as occurs with the ordinary spoilage of **Soy Milk** after long storage in the refrigerator.

Baked Cheeses

(See the section on **Entrees and Nut Main Dishes** for other delicious cheeses, such as **Nuttose**, "**Salmon Loaf**," and **Soy Soufflé**.)

Bold Print indicates items listed in the INDEX

CHEESE

During the fermentation or curing of cheese a mixed group of microorganisms grows in the milk curd. Protein, fat, and carbohydrate are the major nutrients affected during the curing process. The protein portion of cheese is fermented to peptides, amines, indoles, skatole, and ammonia. The fat in cheese is hydrolyzed to irritating fatty acids, butyric, caproic, caprylic, and longer carbon chain fatty acids. The carbohydrate of milk, mainly lactose, is converted to lactic acid by putrefaction. Most of the products of fermentation are toxic and irritating, including the esters, the acids, and certain of the amines, including tyramine and nitrosamine.

A summary of the objectionable features of hard or ripened cheeses includes the following:

1. The putrefactive process results in the production of amines, ammonia, irritating fatty acids (butyric, caproic, caprylic, etc.). The carbohydrate is converted to lactic acid. These are all waste products which cause irritation to nerves and gastro-intestinal tract.
2. Migraine headaches can be caused by tyramine, one of the toxic amines produced in cheese.
3. Certain of the amines can interact with the nitrates present in the stomach to form nitrosamine, a cancer producing agent.
4. An intolerance to lactose, the chief carbohydrate of cheese and milk, is probably the most common food sensitivity in America.
5. Rennet is used in the curdling of milk for cheese making. Rennet is obtained from the whole stomach lining of calves, lambs, kids, or pigs.

Since cottage cheese and cream cheese are not "ripened" it would seem reasonable that these products could safely be used. They are safe, however, only if free from disease-producing organisms, heavy metals, detergents, antibiotics, cancer viruses, and other undesirable substances. In this day of expanding diseases in animals and expanding processes of manufacture and marketing, it is unlikely that any dairy products can be considered safe. Furthermore, rennet, as mentioned in item 5 above, is sometimes used in the production of these cheeses to make a firmer coagulum. Certainly one may object to the use of pig's stomach lining for this purpose.

Cashew Pimiento Cheese

1 c. cashews	¹/₄ c. lemon juice
1 c. water	1 t. salt
¹/₂ c. pimientos	1 t. onion powder
¹/₄ c. yeast flakes	¹/₄ t. garlic powder
¹/₄ c. sesame seed	

Blend all of the ingredients until smooth. To use as a spread bake for 1 hour at 350°. When using for lasagne, macaroni, or pizza just add the blended ingredients to the dish and then bake.

Delicious!

BUTTER
___

Homemade Nut Butters

Use best grade of peanuts, cashews, hazelnuts, walnuts, pecans, almonds, sesame, or sunflower seeds. Roast the nuts or seeds at 275° until light brown. Place 2 cups nuts or seeds in blender and grind to a powder. Then add a little water. Use enough water to make the proper consistency. Use rubber spatula to keep bringing nuts down against blender blades. A little experience will tell you how much water is needed for each type of nut. If you see that too much water has been used for that particular nut, simply add more nuts so that the product will not be liquid. Add salt to taste, about $1/4$ teaspoon to 2 cups. Keeps about one week refrigerated.

Nut Butter

nuts
$1/2$ c. water in blender

$1/4$ t. salt, or more

Add nuts of any kind to blender until the desired consistency of butter is reached. Add flavorings or seasonings as desired, such as vanilla, maple, onion, mint, sage, etc. Store in refrigerator.

Apple Butter

Place **Applesauce** in a large flat pan in the oven to concentrate, while baking other foods. When evaporation has left a thick paste, take up into a storage container. Keeps several weeks in refrigerator. Remove a small amount from storage container as needed. Do not allow storage container to warm up as spoilage is accelerated.

Pear Butter

Use canned pears. Liquefy in blender. Process as for **Apple Butter**. Any canned fruit may be treated in this manner for delicious spreads of low calorie, nutritious quality.

Apricot Butter

$2/3$ c. stewed dried apricots
$2/3$ c. water

honey, if needed for sweetening
1 T. lemon juice

Place ingredients in blender and make a thick paste, using more or less water and apricots. Use as a spread, sandwich filling, or a dessert.

Corn Butter

1 c. corn—fresh, cooked frozen, or
    corn meal mush

$1/2$ t. salt or to taste

Blend smooth with $1/4$ cup water if needed.

Millet, Corn, or Rice Butter

1/4–1/2 c. raw or cooked carrots, optional
1/2–1 1/2 c. water
1/4–1/2 c. coconut, optional

1/2–1 t. salt or more to taste
1 c. hot rice, well cooked (or millet, corn, or corn grits)

Whirl carrots and water in blender, strain and return to blender with remaining ingredients. Blend well. May add garlic or onion, or lemon juice. Dilute for a cream or a salad dressing.

Carob-Tahini Butter or Topping

3/4 c. tahini or **Sesame Butter**
1 T. carob powder

1 T. honey
1/4 c. water

Mix with a fork. Beat in additional water or tahini as needed until consistency of soft butter. Use as spread or topping.

Golden Velvet Butter

3/4 c. cashews, lightly toasted
3 c. water

3 T. agar flakes
1 t. salt, more or less

Gently boil the last 3 ingredients for about 10 minutes. Place all ingredients in blender along with some cooked carrot for yellow color: use about 1/4 to 1 cup. If preferred, use 1/4 to 1 cup cooked yellow corn grits or about 1 teaspoon paprika. Blend for one minute. Chill to set, stir or blenderize to make smooth when ready to serve. Variation: for all or part of the cashews one may substitute cooked whole grains such as rice, millet, or corn grits or may use cooked **Garbanzos** for a delightful spread.

Dessert Topping

1/3 c. white flour
1/3 c. soy flour
1 3/4 c. water or fruit juice
1/2 t. salt

1 T. lemon juice
2–4 T. honey
1 t. vanilla

Dextrinize the flours for 15 minutes at 300°. Put water and flours in blender until smooth. Boil gently for 10 minutes, stirring constantly the first three minutes. Return to blender, add remaining ingredients and blend until smooth. Store in refrigerator up to two weeks. When ready to serve whip with a fork to make smooth again. Serve over cereals, both cooked and dry. Use over waffles, **French Toast** or as a spread for bread. Use over desserts and fruit salads. May add a bit of fruit juice when ready to serve if it congeals too thickly.

BUTTER

Emulsified Nut Butter

Nut Butter is more palatable and more easily eaten and digested if emulsified. To emulsify add cool water to the desired amount of **Nut Butter**, mix thoroughly with a fork, adding the water gradually until mixture is like soft mashed potatoes. Other liquids, such as **Nut Milk**, tomato juice, fruit juice, or a soft banana may be used instead of water. About an equal quantity of water will be required to the quantity of **Nut Butter** used.

Cereal Margarine

1 c. cooked barley **or** rice	$1/2$ c. water, more or less
1 t. **Chicken Style Seasoning**	1–4 T. lemon juice

Whirl together in blender, adding more rice if needed to make quite thick. Try your hand at altering the seasonings and color. Salt to taste like margarine.

EGG SUBSTITUTES

There are several qualities of eggs that need to be replaced in the kitchen. Nutritionally the replacements are easily found. Whole grains, all common varieties of greens, and legumes will supply the nutritional needs usually obtained from eggs. The binding quality of eggs is provided by the yolk and is needed in certain types of loaves and roasts. The binding quality can generally be supplied by flour from any whole grain. Then, there is the leavening agency of the whites of eggs needed in certain quick breads. Generally the use of **Soaked Soybeans** or any kind of legume flour such as soy or garbanzo flour will provide a leavening quality. To find a substitute for egg dishes on the table is also not insurmountable. Use your ingenuity and come up with some simple recipes that will fill an empty spot in the menu where once you used eggs. **Scrambled Tofu** is one such substitute. Following are some substitutes you may wish to try. Determine which quality you need to substitute for, study the recipe and make a selection accordingly.

LEAVENING SUBSTITUTE: Flour made from any bland legume such as garbanzos or soybeans may be used for its slight leavening property. Try about two tablespoons per cup of other flour in the recipe. Use a little extra water as it absorbs water as it cooks. May be used in pancakes.

Mix equal quantities of soy flour and starch. Use about two tablespoons to replace one egg in a recipe. Add some extra water. Two tablespoons almond or cashew butter blended with one tablespoon of lemon juice will replace one egg.

BINDER TO PREVENT BREAKING UP: Any whole grain or legume flour may be used as a binder. Starch gives an unusual binding agency with a crustiness outside. Use about 1–2 tablespoons to replace one egg.

BEATEN-EGG SUBSTITUTE: Use one tablespoon flaxseed to one cup cold water. Soak for one hour. Simmer 20 minutes. Strain and refrigerate until chilled. The liquid forms a gel which beats somewhat like egg white. Will not hold up if heated in the oven.

Soak $1/2$ pound of dried apricots in two cups cold water overnight. Beat thoroughly in a blender, adding water if needed. Strain and chill in refrigerator. Use 1–2 tablespoons to replace one egg in a recipe.

III. DAIRY PRODUCT SUBSTITUTES

Calcium from Common Foods
(Note that milk is not first on the list.)

FOOD	AMOUNT	GRAMS
Collards	1 c.	.498
Dandelions	1 c.	.336
Mustard greens	3/4 c.	.330
Turnip greens, cooked	3/4 c.	.304
Milk	1 c.	.283
Kale	1 c.	.248
Broccoli	1 c.	.245
American cheese	2 T. grated	.175
Baked Beans	1 c.	.146
Figs, dried	4 small	.134
Molasses, Blackstrap	1 T.	.116
Soybeans, dried cooked	3/4 c.	.102
Olives, green	5 small	.075
Cabbage, shredded raw leaf	1 c.	.068
Navy beans, cooked	3/4 c.	.066
String beans, cooked	1/2 c.	.038
Almonds	12–15	.038
Cottage cheese	2 T. rounded	.025

IRON
(Note that milk is a poor source of iron.)

FOOD	AMOUNT	MG.
Mustard greens, cooked	1/3 c.	5.6
Turnip greens, cooked	1/3 c.	3.5
Navy beans, cooked	1/2 c.	3.1
Swiss chard, cooked	1/2 c.	3.1
Lentils, cooked	1/2 c.	2.9
Soybeans, cooked	1/2 c.	2.5
Apricots, dried	4–6 halves	2.3
Loganberries, fresh	1/2–3/4 c.	2.1
Molasses	1 T.	1.9
Prunes, dried	4–5	1.8
Peaches, dried	2 halves	1.8
Egg	1	1.6
Sweet potato, baked	1 large	1.4
Avocado	1/2 medium	1.4
White potato	1 small	1.1
Bread, whole wheat	1 slice	0.9
Milk, whole	1 c.	0.2

Thiamine

FOOD	AMOUNT	MG.
GRAINS		
Rye, whole, cooked	3/4 c.	0.47
Wheat germ	1 T.	0.2–0.4
Rice, brown, cooked	1/2 c.	0.29
Sweet corn	1/2 c.	0.20
Whole wheat, cooked	3/4 c.	0.15–0.198
Rolled oats, cooked	2/3 c.	0.104–0.231
Whole wheat bread	1 slice	0.072–0.12
LEGUMES		
Split peas	1/2 c.	0.87
Soybeans, dried, cooked	1/2 c.	0.36
Soy flour	1/2 c.	0.3–0.6
Peas, fresh	1/2 c.	0.27–0.495
Lima beans, cooked	1/2 c.	0.25–0.35
FRUIT		
Avocado	1/2 medium	0.1–0.2
Prunes	4–5 medium	0.088–0.113
NUTS		
Brazil nuts	2 medium	0.158
GREENS		
Collards	1/2 c.	0.22
Turnip greens	1/2 c.	0.138–0.18
MISCELLANEOUS		
Brewer's yeast	1 T.	0.5–0.8
Milk	1 c.	0.096–0.156

Bold Print indicates items listed in the INDEX

III. DAIRY PRODUCT SUBSTITUTES

FOOD VALUE CHARTS

Comparative Values

FOOD	AMOUNT	CALCIUM Mg.	PROTEIN Gms.	RIBOFLAVIN Mg.	CALORIES
Soybeans	1 c.	132	21.0	0.18	99
Milk	1 c.	288	8.5	0.48	166
Lentils	1 c.	36	15.0	0.12	210
Kale	1 c.	248	4.2	0.24	35
Dandelions	1 c.	336		0.22	40
Figs	10	270	7.0	0.25	395
Collards	1 c.	498	7.8	0.48	80
Almonds	12	38	2.8	0.10	90
Baked Beans	1 c.	146	15.0	0.08	280
Blackstrap	1 T.	116	0	0.05	43
Mustard	1 c.	330	3.6	0.27	33
Rutabagas	1 c.	88	1.2	0.12	52
Turnip greens	1 c.	376	4.2	0.60	44

Food Sources of the Vitamins

VITAMIN	SOURCES
A	Green and yellow vegetables and fruits.
B_1	(Thiamine) Whole grains, legumes, nuts, greens.
B_2	(Riboflavin) Greens, wheat, vegetables.
B_3	(Niacin) Whole grains, nuts.
B_6	(Pyridoxine) Wheat, nuts, legumes, cabbage, bananas. (Pantothenic acid) Legumes, wheat. (Biotin) Legumes. (Folic acid) Green vegetables, wheat. (Choline) Whole grains.
C	Greens, peppers, citrus fruits, cabbage, tomatoes, potatoes.
D	Sunshine: A fair-skinned person needs only a 6″ square of skin exposed daily to the sun for 1 hour. The darker the skin the longer the exposure needed.
E	Vegetable oils, whole grains, vegetables.
K	Cabbage, cauliflower, spinach.

Bold Print indicates items listed in the INDEX

IV. DESSERTS

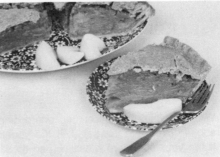

IV. DESSERTS

INTRODUCTION

BASIC RULES IN CHOOSING DESSERTS

When the quality of home cooking reaches the level that ordinary breads are relished and fruits are enjoyed in their natural goodness, there will be little need for unwholesome cakes, pastries, and sugary snacks.

1. When choosing a dessert the entire dinner must be considered: the **Main Dish**, the cooked dish, and the salad. If the vegetables are starchy the dessert must be light. If the vegetables are mostly green then the dessert can be more filling. It is a good rule to make desserts so that each serving contains around 1 teaspoon of sugar. Keeping the sweetener low allows for some sugars to be eaten in other dishes, without running the risk that the quantity of sugars that the body can handle without suffering damage will be exceeded.

2. Do not serve the meal in courses, but put all the food, including the dessert, on the table at once. The diners may then make a more judicious choice of the amount of food to eat. Serving in courses promotes overeating.

3. Almost everybody now recognizes that rich and heavy desserts are undesirable, causing stomach irritation, mental dullness, and overweight. The simpler the dessert, the more satisfying and healthful.

4. Other good rules are: Do not serve too much to eat, and do not have too many heavy starches or other concentrated foods at a meal. The sections on **Fruit Meal Desserts** and **Fruit Salads** should give the cook some ideas on how the various fruits may be served with meals all year round. Fruits are especially healthful when they are in season. Fruit may comprise a whole dinner with side dishes of **Soy Yogurt** or **Sour Cream** and **Bread**. Nothing is more delightful to serve out-of-doors, or more satisfying, than such a dinner on a warm summer day.

5. Omit nuts, seeds, wheat germ, and coconut if your diet is oil-free.

For other simple desserts try several of the fine recipes in the sections on **Breakfasts**; **Breads**; **Fruit Salads**; and **Cereal, Waffle, and Dessert Toppings, Spreads**.

Bold Print indicates items listed in the INDEX

Wheat Germ Pie Crust

Moisten pie pan with water. Sprinkle about $1/4''$ layer of wheat germ onto it. Fill with custard or filling. Bake. Variations: use corn meal, bread crumbs, or flaked dry cereal.

Crisp Topping
(Pie Crust)

3 c. oats, rolled	1 t. vanilla
$1/4$–$1/2$ t. salt	2–4 T. honey
$1^1/_2$ c. fruit sauce or water	$1/4$ c. nuts, optional

Let this crisp cook over any fruit or berry filling. Bake at 375° for 45 minutes. Use as little water as possible as the more water used the more likely it is to be hard. During the last 10 minutes of baking, baste once or twice with fruit juice, if desired, to soften.

Orange Peel Topping

Preserve the peelings from unsprayed oranges when they are available. Dry in a warm oven. (May place peelings in oven immediately after removing a baked dish. Turn oven off and allow peelings to dry.) Grind dry peelings in seed mill or blender. Store in tightly covered jar in refrigerator or freezer. We lay in a year's supply when unsprayed oranges are available.

Granola Pie Crust

Moisten pie pan with water. Sprinkle about $1/4''$ layer of Granola or ground granola on to it. Fill with custard or other pie filling. Variations: Use toasted bread crumbs or flake dry cereal.

Almond Pie Crust

$1^1/_2$ c. almonds or other nuts	$1/2$ c. unbleached white flour
$3/4$ c. whole wheat flour	$1/2$ t. salt

Grind almonds finely (about to butter) in seed mill or blender. Mix the dry ingredients with the ground almonds and add $1/3$ cup or more of warm water. Divide in half.

Roll out between layers of plastic wrap. Makes two pie crusts. Bake at 350° until golden brown.

Bold Print indicates items listed in the INDEX

IV. DESSERTS

Ground Seed Topping

Preserve seed from all vegetables such as cantaloupe, squash, or other melons having a soft enough seed shell to eat comfortably. Dry in oven and lightly toast while baking other foods. Grind in a seed mill to a fine powder. Use as toppings for fruit or as a garnish over whipped soy cream or stewed fruit.

Other Topping Suggestions

See the INDEX for several carob recipes in this book such as **Carob Pudding** and **Carob Sauce** which can be used as toppings or icings. **Coconut Gravy**; **Basic Gravy** and **Custard**; **Vanilla Sauce**; **Fruit Sauce**, **Puddings**, **Custard** are all toppings listed in the INDEX which are suitable for desserts.

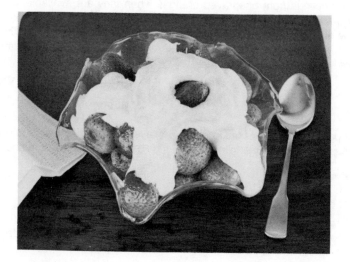

Bold Print indicates items listed in the INDEX

IV. DESSERTS

Fruit Kisses

2 c. mixed, ground, dried fruit
$^1/_2$ c. ground pecan meats

2 T. lemon juice

Mix and press into a roll. Wrap in plastic film. Refrigerate overnight. Slice in $^1/_4$" slices with sharp knife. May be made into small balls and rolled in carob powder or unsweetened coconut.

Seedy Morsel

Chop in electric food mill 5 tablespoons sunflower seed; 5 tablespoons pumpkin seed; coarsely. Mix with 6 tablespoons macaroon coconut, 5 tablespoons carob powder, and 4 tablespoons honey. Add barely enough water to make a dry paste. Make $^3/_4$" balls and roll in macaroon coconut. Makes 56 balls.

Seed Mounds

2 c. nuts, seeds, or coconut,
lightly toasted

$^1/_3$ c. honey
$^1/_8$ t. salt

Boil honey and salt until a drop forms a soft ball in cold water. Add nuts and mix well. Drop by tablespoons onto a platter. Makes about 16 to 20 mounds. Each mound contains 1 ounce of nuts and 1 teaspoon honey when 16 mounds are made from the recipe.

Bold Print indicates items listed in the INDEX

IV. DESSERTS

Carob Custard

$^1/_2$ c. pecans
4 c. water
$^1/_2$ t. salt

$^1/_4$ c. carob
$^1/_4$ c. honey **or** Karo
6 T. starch

Blend ingredients together until nuts are smooth. Heat until thick, stirring constantly. Pour into custard cups, sprinkle with coconut and serve with **Maranola**. **Serves 6**.

Carob Pudding

3 T. starch
2 T. soy flour
3 T. carob powder
$^1/_4$ t. salt

$^1/_4$ c. Karo
$1^3/_4$ c. **Soy or Nut Milk**
2 t. vanilla
1 c. whole, lightly toasted peanuts

Mix all ingredients except last two and cook 5 minutes, stirring constantly. Add vanilla and peanuts and pour into molds to cool. Serve with a dessert topping. May be used with a fruit meal. Serves 6, $^1/_2$ cup each.

Baked Sweet Potatoes

sweet potatoes in 1–2″ chunks
water

pecans, chopped
salt

Use one medium size, well-baked sweet potato for each serving. Mix with sufficient water to make the consistency of very soft, mashed potatoes, but leave some chunks. May need to use a potato masher on larger chunks. Add 1 tablespoon pecans for each serving. Salt to taste. Bake at 350° for 1–2 hours, the longer baked the sweeter it gets. Serve with **Coconut Gravy**.

Sweet Potato Crisp

Use the above recipe for **Baked Sweet Potatoes** and cover with the **Crisp Topping** recipe given in this section. Bake at 300° to 325° for $1^1/_2$ hours.

Cantaloupe Cream

1 cantaloupe
$^1/_4$ c. Soyagen powder

pinch of salt

Peel cantaloupe, remove seeds (saving them for making **Seed Powder**) and whirl in blender with other ingredients until smooth. Serve with sprigs of mint. Serves 4–6.

Bold Print indicates items listed in the INDEX

IV. DESSERTS

Sweet Potato Pudding

5 c. sweet potatoes
2 T. honey, optional
$\frac{1}{2}$ t. salt

$\frac{1}{2}$ t. vanilla
2 t. coriander
$\frac{1}{4}$ t. orange extract

Mash together until smooth, using a potato masher. Dip into 6 custard cups and bake for 30–45 minutes. Variations: Use also as a pie. Place in unbaked pie shell. Bake at 350° for $1\frac{1}{2}$ hours.

Pumpkin Pie or Pudding

$3\frac{1}{4}$ c. cooked pumpkin, mashed smooth
2 c. soy or nut milk
$\frac{1}{4}$ c. starch
$\frac{1}{4}$ c. honey
$\frac{1}{2}$ c. date **or** raw sugar

1 T. vanilla
1 T. coriander
$1\frac{1}{2}$ T. molasses
$\frac{1}{2}$ t. salt

Blend smooth. Pour into two unbaked pie shells. Bake at 425° for 15 minutes, then at 250° for $1\frac{1}{4}$ hours. Chill to set.

Sweet Potato Pie

1 c. unbleached white flour **or** oat flour
4 c. drained canned **or** peeled baked
    sweet potatoes
2 t. vanilla

2 T. honey, optional
1 t. salt
1 c. water

Stir together, mashing potatoes or blending with the water to make smooth, or leaving chunky as desired. Pour into floured baking dish. Bake at 350° for 30–60 minutes.

Chiffon Pumpkin Pie

2–3 c. winter squash, cooked
$\frac{2}{3}$ c. water, if needed
$\frac{1}{4}$ t. salt
2 T. agar

1 c. water
$\frac{1}{3}$ c. Soyagen powder
$\frac{2}{3}$ c. water

Put last two items in blender and whirl. Pour into large mixing bowl. Put squash in blender with salt and up to $\frac{1}{3}$ cup water if needed to turn blender. Whirl until smooth. Boil agar and 1 cup water for 1–2 minutes. Stir into Soyagen mixture. Add squash and swirl once with a spatula, but leave partly unmixed to give marbleized effect. Pour up into tall, stem glasses or **Pie Crust**. Top with grated orange peel or nuts. Serves 6 or 7, about $\frac{1}{2}$ cup each.

Bold Print indicates items listed in the INDEX

IV. DESSERTS

Sweet Potato Cakes

6 baked sweet potatoes
water
$^1/_3$ c. shredded coconut, optional

2 T. flour
1 T. grated orange peel
salt to taste

Peel potatoes and use a potato masher to make a very thick paste with water. Add remaining ingredients. Form into small cakes and bake at 350° until brown crust forms. Serve with **Basic Gravy**. About 6 servings.

Goober Pudding

$3^1/_2$ c. water
$^1/_2$ c. unbleached white flour
2–3 T. honey

$^1/_3$ t. salt
$^1/_2$ c. toasted peanuts **or** other nuts
1 t. vanilla

Put the water, honey, salt, and peanuts in a blender and whirl until smooth. Add the flour. Whirl to distribute well. Cook for 10 minutes, stirring constantly for the first 3 minutes until thick, then reducing heat to a slow boil. Serves 4, about $^1/_2$ cup each.

Bold Print indicates items listed in the INDEX

Rhubarb Pie

2 qts. canned sweet potatoes and liquid
$1/2$ c. honey
$1/2$ t. salt

2 c. water
1 c. tapioca
$3^1/_2$ qts. chopped rhubarb

Soak tapioca in water for 5 minutes. Mix with rhubarb and bring to a boil. Add remaining ingredients. Pour into a floured casserole and bake for $1^1/_2$ hours at 350°.

Carrot Pie

$1^1/_2$ c. **Soy Milk**
2 c. cooked carrots
3 T. soy **or** oat flour
2 T. honey

$1/2$ t. vanilla
$2^1/_2$ T. starch
$1/2$ t. salt

Whirl in blender. Pour into baked **Pie Crust**. Bake at 300° for 1 hour. Cool and serve. Variation: Use winter squash for carrots.

Creamed Artichokes

4 c. water
$1/3$ c. tapioca
$2/3$ c. nuts
$1/2$ t. salt

$1/4$ c. honey
1 t. vanilla
2 c. Jerusalem artichokes

Chop Jerusalem artichokes into $1/2$" cubes. Cook about 20 minutes or until tender. Set aside to cool. Put 2 cups water in a stewer with the tapioca to soak 15 minutes. Boil for 5 minutes, stirring occasionally. Remove from heat. Meanwhile, put remaining 2 cups water in blender with nuts, salt, honey, and vanilla. Blend until smooth milk is obtained. Pour into tapioca with artichokes. Cool in refrigerator. Becomes slightly thick. Garnish top with fresh chopped mint. Serves 8–10. Variation: Substitute sweet potatoes for artichokes.

Bold Print indicates items listed in the INDEX

IV. DESSERTS

Fruit Pie

4 c. sweet fruit **or** berries
1–4 T. honey, if needed
1–2 T. starch

$^1/_3$ c. water, if needed in blender
$^1/_8$ t. salt
2 T. lemon juice (omit for tart fruit)

Place about $^1/_2$ cup fruit or more in **Pie Crust** or atop a thick layer of **Maranola** or **Granola** in a baking dish. Set aside. Blend rest of fruit with honey, water, starch, and salt. Boil until thickened. Add lemon juice. Cool slightly and spoon over whole fruit. Use as breakfast main dish with **Coconut Cream**. Serves 4, 1 cup each.

Lemon Custard

1 c. water
2 c. fresh **Orange Sauce or** pineapple
    juice

juice and rind of 1 lemon
2 T. honey
$^1/_4$ c. starch

Put whole lemon, quartered to remove seeds, into blender with all ingredients until ground fine. Bring this mixture to a boil and simmer about 2 minutes. Stir constantly. Pour into serving dishes. Decorate with pecans, a date, or a few raisins. Use also as pie filling. Serves 6, $^1/_2$ cup each. Variation: Use 3 oranges, peeled, and quartered to remove seeds, instead of orange juice. Placed peeled oranges in blender with lemon to be chopped.

Orchard Apple Pie

3 c. grated apples
2 c. pineapple juice

$3^1/_2$ T. tapioca or arrowroot powder

Blend pineapple juice and thickening agent. Boil, stirring constantly to thicken. Cool and mix with the grated apples. Put into a baked pie crust and serve cold. Variations: Mix raisins or other dried fruit in filling. Cover with unsweetened coconut.

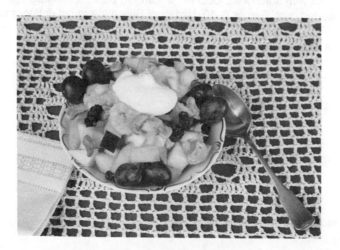

IV. DESSERTS

Ambrosia

3 large oranges
2 ripe bananas, sliced

$1/2$ c. coconut, unsweetened, grated
3 T. **Grated Orange Rind**

Peel, quarter, and remove seed from oranges. Blend in blender until fine. Mix all ingredients. Garnish with mint sprigs or sweet basil. Serves 5–6.

DESSERTS

We have become a nation of metabolic cripples because of our overuse of sugar, animal products, oil, salt and other rich foods. Many suffer from dizziness, fatigue, excessive hunger, allergies, nervousness, overweight, hypertension, and a host of other symptoms of metabolic disorders. The imbalance of the biochemistry caused by the imbalance of the dietary elements is the cause of much suffering. The high fat content of the diet is particularly damaging. Fats are handled in a special way by the digestive tract, even to the point of being carried from the intestinal tract mainly by a special vessel system, the lymphatic vessels. If fats were released readily from the stomach to the intestinal tract, the vessels would be overpowered, too much fat would enter the blood, and the circulation would be hindered or even stopped.

Too much sugar similarly burdens the blood. The blood is actually made syrupy by much sugar. Secondarily, other body fluids are made heavy, such as the fluids of the brain, eyes, joints, and bursae. The sluggishness of the entire body brought on by too much sugar causes disease. All tissues of the body are affected.

Lemon Cream Pie

$1/3$ c. coconut, ground fine
1 c. pineapple juice
3 T. lemon juice

$1/2$ t. lemon rind **or** extract
$1/4$ t. salt
6 T. corn starch or arrowroot

Blend. Stir into 2 cups boiling pineapple juice. Continue stirring until thick. Pour into baked pie shell. May use granola crust. Decorate with mint leaves or nuts.

Bold Print indicates items listed in the INDEX

IV. DESSERTS

Baked Apples

baking apples
dates

sprinkle of salt

Wash and core 1 apple for each person. Place 1 date in the empty center. Sprinkle very lightly with salt. Place in a baking pan with a little water in bottom of pan. Bake about 40 to 60 minutes at 350°.

Berry Pie

4 c. berries, any kind
Maranola or Granola
2 c. fruit juice **or** water

$1/4$ c. starch
1–4 T. Karo **or** honey
$1/8$ t. salt

Cook last four ingredients until starch is thick, stirring constantly. Cool slightly. Add berries and pour into a dish lined with **Maranola**. Top with more **Maranola**, using about $1/2$ to $2/3$ cup per person to be served. Use as a **Main Dish** at **Breakfast** or as a fruit dessert. About 4 servings.

Banana Cream Pie

4 c. **Nut or Soy Milk**
2 T. honey
$1/2$ c. unsweetened coconut, optional
$1/2$ c. starch

$1/4$ t. salt
1 t. vanilla
4 ripe bananas

Put the first six ingredients in a saucepan and stir constantly while cooking until thick. Mash two bananas and add to mixture. Do not cook bananas. Slice the other bananas and add. Pour into baked **Pie Crust** and chill until set. May use **Granola** for crust and topping, making individual servings in custard cups. Serves 6–8.

Banana Cream Toast

3 c. **Soy or Nut Milk**
$3/4$ c. flour

$1/4$ t. salt, heaping
4 bananas

Blend milk, flour, and salt, heat to thicken while stirring, then gently simmer for about 10 minutes. Return to blender with the bananas and blend until smooth. Serve on toast, or dip **Melba Toast** into mixture and serve on plates. Top with a sprinkle of chopped nuts, if desired. Serves 8.

Bold Print indicates items listed in the INDEX

IV. DESSERTS

Prune Cake

24 prunes
8 slices whole wheat bread

1 t. vanilla
fruit juice

Soak dried prunes overnight. Cover with $1/2''$ of water and cook until soft with a few slices of lemon or orange added to give them flavor. Put the prunes and cooking water through a colander to separate the pits and make a thin puree. Flavor with vanilla. Line a square cake pan with 4 slices of bread. Pour enough fruit juice to moisten the bread, and cover with half of the prune pulp about $1/2''$ deep. Repeat the process. Put into the oven at 350° for 25 minutes so it will set. Cool, cut into squares, and serve with a teaspoon of **Whipped Topping** on each serving. Good as a main dish for breakfast. Serves 4–6.

Plumped Prunes

Select a good grade of large prunes. Place loosely in a jar and cover with hot water. Leave overnight or until as soft as fresh prunes. Store in refrigerator and have ready when needed on short notice.

Stewed Dried Prunes
May use apricots or other dried fruit

Cover with water, and let soak several hours, or until sufficient water has been absorbed to make them soft. Simmer slowly until thoroughly done. Thicken the water with a little starch. Add Karo or honey to sweeten apricots if necessary. Use as a dessert or as a topping for cereals or dessert breads.

Apple Crisp

6–8 large apples

1 **Crisp Topping** recipe

Slice applies into shallow pan. Spread **Crisp Topping** evenly over apples. Bake at 375° until golden brown, about 45 minutes.

Serving Suggestions: Use as a breakfast meal with a topping of hot **Applesauce**, or as a dessert with topping of soy cream or **Whipped Topping**. Yield: 8–10 servings.

Swedish Grape Creme

Heat in saucepan 1 quart of fresh or home-canned scuppernongs or grapes. Separate pulp and skins. Place pulp in blender at lowest speed for just long enough to separate seeds from pulp. Remove seeds in a colander. Blend skins and pulp until fine. Put skins, pulp, $1/2$ cup honey, and 3 tablespoons tapioca in saucepan. Cook over medium heat, stirring occasionally. Pour into 4–6 sherbet glasses. Cool in refrigerator. Serve with **Nut Cream**.

IV. DESSERTS

Apple Lauf

4 diced or shredded apples
grated rind of 1 lemon

juice of 1 orange
2 c. fluffy bread crumbs

Mix the diced apples with rind and juice. Sprinkle baking dish with a layer of crumbs, then a layer of apple mixture. Continue until all are used, topping with crumbs. Bake at 350° for 30 to 40 minutes. If it seems a bit dry, cover during baking. Serve hot with **Nut Cream**. Serves 2–3.

Apple Pudding

4 c. sweet apples
1 lemon, quartered
$^3/_4$ c. raisins
1 T. starch

1 c. water
2 c. **Melba Toast** crumbs
$^1/_8$ t. salt

Place all ingredients in blender except apples and crumbs and liquefy. Use more water if necessary to make a thin mixture. In shallow baking dish place alternating layers of crumbs and chopped apples. Pour raisin mixture over and bake at 350° for 45 to 60 minutes. Serve hot or cold. Yield: 4 servings.

Arkansas Puddin'

4 c. **Granola**
4 c. **Applesauce**

roasted pecan halves **or** other nuts
for garnish

Mix **Granola** and **Applesauce**, making quite a soupy mixture. Allow to sit overnight for **Granola** to absorb the fluid of the **Applesauce**. Next morning garnish with nuts and heat in oven if desired. Serve with **Whipped Topping** or **Fruit Sauce**.

Carob Drink

2 c. **Soy or Nut Milk**
$^1/_4$ t. vanilla

2–4 T. carob
pinch of salt

Place all ingredients in blender until smooth. Serve hot or cold. Yield: 4 small servings. Variation: Add 3 dates or 1 banana.

Prune Whip

1 c. **Nut Milk**
3 c. prunes **or** other dried fruit

1 T. sesame seed
1 T. carob

Whirl in a blender until smooth. Put in custard cups and chill. Sprinkle with more toasted sesame seed. Yield: 8–10 servings.

Bread Pudding

15 slices bread, cubed
3 c. water
1/3 c. **Soy Base**
3/4 t. salt

1 1/2 c. raisins **or** 6 small apples,
    chopped
1 t. vanilla
1 T. **Grated Orange Rind**
3 T. honey

Put all the ingredients except bread in blender. Blend coarsely and add to the cubed bread. Bake in a pretty casserole at 350° for 1 hour. Served as a dessert cold and sliced with **Whipped Topping**, or hot as a breakfast dish with **Fruit Sauce**. If apples are used, may add 2–4 tablespoons Karo or honey. About 8 servings.

Hominy Pie

6 c. hot, salted **Corn Grits**
1/4 c. Karo

5 c. chopped, drained, canned
    fruit, pears good

Mix all ingredients while grits are hot. Pour into casserole or dessert cups. Allow to cool to congeal. Add desired topping and bake 15 to 20 minutes at 400°. Serves 6 if used as breakfast cereal. Serves 12 as dessert. Use a topping of nuts, coconut, **Grated Orange Rind** or **Granola**.

Fruit Squares

2 T. honey
1/3 c. water
1 c. flour
1 t. salt
1 1/2 c. quick oats
1/2 c. oat flour (grind rolled oats in blender)

1 c. dates **or** raisins
1 c. water
1 t. lemon juice
1/2 t. vanilla
2 T. starch
1/8 t. salt

Mix in separate bowls the first two and the next four items, then combine and crumble together. Prepare filling by mixing last six ingredients and boiling until soft. Press half of the crumbly mixture on bottom of floured pan. Spread filling over that, and cover with rest of crumbly mixture. Bake at 375° for 40 minutes, until browned. Cool. Wet the top layer by spooning 3/4 cup pineapple juice over top. Cover pan and set in refrigerator overnight. Cut 6–8 squares. Variation: Prepare filling from 2 cups crushed, unsweetened pineapple, canned pears, or apples instead of dates and water.

Bold Print indicates items listed in the INDEX

IV. DESSERTS

Steamed Irish Raisin Pudding

$1^1/_2$ c. **Nut Milk**
$1^1/_2$ c. plumped raisins
$1^1/_2$ c. whole wheat flour
$^1/_2$ t. salt
3 T. sorghum **or** honey

$^1/_4$ t. coriander
1 T. grated lemon rind
$1^1/_2$ c. bread crumbs
1 c. grated, peeled apple

Combine ingredients and turn into well floured 2 quart tube mold or fruit juice can. Steam for 2 hours (see **Covered Steamer**). Cool and unmold. Slice and serve with **Nut Cream** or **Applesauce**. Yield: 6 servings. Variation: Try fresh cooked hot **Millet**, or leftover **Rice** instead of bread crumbs.

Baked Bananas Hawaii

Peel $^1/_2$ to 1 banana per person and put in well floured baking dish. Drip honey, if glaze desired, over top and bake at 450° until puffed and brown, about 10 minutes. (May mix orange or lemon juice with honey and dip bananas in mixture before baking.)

Banana Popsicle

Peel banana. Cut in half crosswise. Put on a popsicle stick. Cover with date butter (4 dates heated with 4 teaspoons water) and roll in coconut or cereal flakes. Put in freezer and freeze. Take out of freezer a little before serving.

Bold Print indicates items listed in the INDEX

Pineapple Pudding

4 c. unsweetened pineapple juice
$^1/_3$ c. starch or $^3/_4$ c. farina
$^1/_4$ t. mint flavoring, optional

1 c. crushed unsweetened pineapple, drained
$^1/_2$ t. salt

Bring 3 cups juice to rolling boil. Mix starch with 1 cup juice and add gradually, stirring constantly. Add remaining ingredients, pour into dessert cups. Chill and serve with topping of coconut, chopped nuts, or **Whipped Topping**. Yield: 8–10 servings.

Banana Nut Cake

8–10 slices **Zwieback**
2 c. fruit juice **or** water
$^1/_2$ c. Karo **or** honey
1 t. salt
1 t. vanilla
1 c. mashed bananas

1 T. orange **or** lemon rind
2 c. flour
1 t. coriander, ground
$^1/_4$ c. wheat bran **or** germ
$^1/_2$ c. nuts

Omit the last two items on strictly oil free diets. Chop the **Zwieback** to $^1/_3$″ squares. Mix the last five ingredients. Add the remaining ingredients which have been stirred together, except for the **Zwieback**, which is added last to give the proper texture to the cake. The **Zwieback** squares should not become so limp in the dough that they collapse or lose their enclosed air spaces. Pour into 2 cake pans 1″ deep. Bake for 35 minutes until golden brown at 350°. Cool on towels. Variation: Use 1 cup crushed pineapple or raisins for bananas. Ice with **Carob Sauce** at the time of serving. Yield: 10 to 12 servings.

Uncooked Fruit Cake

1 c. raisins, ground
1 c. dates, chopped
2 c. dried fruit, chopped, any kind
$^3/_4$ c. water

1 c. whole wheat bread crumbs
1 c. fruit juice **or** nectar
1 c. sunflower seed **or** nuts (omit on oil-free diets)

Soak the dried fruits in the water and fruit juice for 2 hours. Add crumbs and seed. Pack into floured mold. Set for one or more days in refrigerator. Unmold, slice, and serve with **Soy Yogurt**.

Bold Print indicates items listed in the INDEX

IV. DESSERTS

Kumquat Jelly

2 c. sliced kumquats
2 c. unsweetened canned apples
$1/4$ c. water

1 T. starch
1 T. honey

Mix ingredients. Bring to a boil, stirring constantly. Boil gently for 30 minutes. Serve hot over toast or banana nut bread. Store in refrigerator up to 2 weeks.

Apple Leather

Blend 1 quart of unsweetened apples, canned or fresh, until smooth. Pour about $1/4$" thick into a large flat plan which has been lined with plastic wrap. Dry in air or slightly warm oven for 1–2 days. Peel up from pan and cut in squares with kitchen shears. Serve at the end of a fruit meal as an unusual dessert. Try this same technique with pears, tomatoes, peaches, watermelon, or any other fruit or succulent vegetable. Store in plastic bags. Keeps indefinitely if stored airtight. Good camping food as it is lightweight and filling.

Ice Cream (Fruit Smoothie)

Peel and freeze bananas or other fruit.

Put 4 inch pieces in the blender with $1/4$ c. water or juice. Blend smooth.

Add other fruits as desired, or extracts such as strawberries, blueberries, pears, vanilla, maple, and almond. May add nuts such as walnuts, pecans, cashews, and coconut. Serve in tall glasses.

Millet Pudding

1 c. hot cooked millet (i.e. 1 c. dry millet,
    $2^1/2$ c. water, $1/2$ t. salt)
2 c. pineapple juice
$1/4$ t. salt

1 t. vanilla
1 T. cashews **or** 2 T. coconut,
    optional

Blend smooth, pour into serving dish and chill. Layer with fruit if desired, such as pineapple, bananas, peaches, berries, or grapes.

Decorate with fruit, nuts, mint leaves, etc. May add one of the following while blending to change flavor or color:

2 T. carob + $1/2$ t. lemon or orange extract or 1 T. rind.

Bold Print indicates items listed in the INDEX

V. ENTREES & NUT MAIN DISHES

V. ENTREES AND NUT MAIN DISHES

<u>INTRODUCTION</u>

PROTEINS AND B-VITAMINS

Entrees should supply either a good quality or a good quantity of protein, and generous amounts of B-vitamins. Since the body requires a steady supply of proteins for growth and repair, and the mind must have readily available B-vitamins for proper thinking and steady nerves, our Divine Creator has put these two important nutrients in a wide variety of foods. Vegetables, fruits, and whole grains supply all the food elements needed to maintain health. If one is concerned about vitamin B_{12} intake, he may easily supplement his diet with certain food yeasts which have been produced in such a way as to contain this vitamin, or with commercially available B_{12}. One can thus maintain the advantages of avoiding animal products and still get sufficient B_{12} to meet the National Research Council recommendation.

Obtain as wide a variety of unrefined foods as possible to give the body an exposure to trace minerals and/or micronutrients whose existence may not yet be understood.

Nuts and seeds are a pleasant luxury in the diet and are not nutritionally essential. For those who must fashion an oil-free diet, omit them from each recipe. The greens have such a good quality of protein that their presence in a meal in generous amounts makes the protein content of other foods of less importance. It is not necessary to use concentrated nutrients to prepare the main dishes, such as adding concentrated proteins or vitamins to the dish, merely to enrich the food. Concentrated nutrients should be used sparingly. Remember that the primary rule in nutrition is a wide variety.

LEGUMES AND WHOLE GRAINS—GOOD COMBINATION

The casserole is an easy and attractive way to serve a main dish. Many of the entrees presented in this chapter can be served this way. Some of these dishes utilize leftovers; and best of all, many may be made ahead of time to heat up or bake at the last minute. In our hurried lives every cook wants the best possible food with a minimum of work and fuss. Garbanzo, lentil, and other bean dishes are fine for small or large banquets. Their flavors are enjoyed by everyone and their food value is excellent. When used with whole grain bread, dumplings, rice, or pastas they provide a fine quality protein of high biologic value.

CHANGES IN STARCH BY COOKING

Some foods are more nourishing if they have a short cooking period. The succulent vegetables such as summer squash fall in this category. Other foods do not release to us their nutrients until they have been well cooked. Grains, legumes, and very starchy vegetables such as carrots and potatoes are in this group. Unmilled grains need several hours cooking.

Raw starch granules in grains and starchy vegetables are surrounded by a fibrous skeleton which holds the minerals and proteins. The action of heat and water softens and ruptures the fibrous shell, and breaks the long chain starch molecules to short chain dextrins. The minerals and vitamins are released from the fibrous shells and are available for absorption from the intestinal tract. Microscopically one can see first the formation of smaller units, then the complete dissolution of the starch grains. It seems wise to eat the heaviest carbohydrates at the first of a meal while the concentration of salivary amylase is still high.

PASTAS

To most people pasta means nothing more than macaroni and cheese, or spaghetti with tomato sauce. Actually a vast array of main dishes can be made with **Pastas**. Combine spaghetti with steamed, sauteed vegetables, or with fruit and nuts, or just plain garlic and plenty of freshly chopped onions. Use your ingenuity to create your own dishes.

Be careful not to have too much pasta for the sauce. The pasta must be well mixed so that each piece glistens with sauce. The use of whole grain **Pastas** by Italians is credited with giving them a very low incidence of both heart trouble and cancer. The fiber of whole grains is very effective in keeping the cholesterol low and in maintaining good bowel health, free from ulcers, diverticula, polyps, and cancer.

COOKING INSTRUCTIONS

Macaroni and **Spaghetti** are added to actively boiling salted water, 6–8 cups of water to 8 ounces of the pasta. It is cooked from 15 to 20 minutes, depending on its thickness. After 15 minutes test it for doneness. It should not be cooked until it is mushy, but removed from the fire while it is still "chewy" or *al dente*, as this state is called by the Italians. Boiling time is cut down several minutes if **Pastas** are to be combined with other foods and baked in the oven.

NUTS AS MAIN DISHES

Nuts are concentrated foods and should be used in small quantities. No more than $1/6$ to $1/10$ of any dish should be of nuts. They should never be eaten between meals. Frying nuts or roasting in oil makes them harder to digest. If eaten fresh or slightly roasted, they are easily digested. Commercially obtained raw nuts should be sterilized in the oven at 300° for 15 minutes. This practice is especially important for nuts obtained from foreign countries. Peanuts and other legumes have many properties in common with nuts.

DANGEROUS FOODS

Because of certain serious and life-threatening diseases of animals, all animal products carry some risk in their use. Certain of these diseases are so malignant that all would be well advised to avoid risk entirely. Luncheon and variety meats such as salami, sausage, frankfurters, and liverwurst fall in this category. They are high in saturated fats. Further, they are often composed of refuse meats that could not be marketed whole because of their disgusting appearance or unwholesome properties. Ground, seasoned and colored, they are disguised.

Since there is no difficulty in obtaining a complete array of proteins, carbohydrates, calories, minerals, vitamins, fiber, water, and fat from a dietary that does not include any animal products, we are presenting this section for those who want an experience in eating that will be simultaneously interesting, tasty, nutritious **and** harmless. For us, the experiment with vegetarian cookery can easily be termed "high adventure."

LEGUMES

Cooked Garbanzos
Mexican Chick Peas

Since garbanzos require long cooking, it is wise to cook a large batch and freeze a portion. Sort peas and wash. Soak 3–4 cups garbanzos covered with 2″ of cold water overnight. Add 2 teaspoons salt. Cook in pressure cooker at 5–10 pounds for 1–2 hours or in regular saucepan 6–8 hours. They are now ready for use in your favorite recipe.

Garbanzos

8 c. **Garbanzos, Cooked**
pimientos, chopped
1–2 c. water

$^1/_3$ c. rolled oats
1 t. garlic powder
2 t. salt

Whirl the last four ingredients in the blender until smooth and add to the garbanzos. Cook for 15 minutes using chopped pimientos for color and flavor. Serves 8–10.

Garbanzos Mexican Style

4 c. **Cooked Garbanzos**
1 onion **or** green pepper, minced
2 T. syrup **or** molasses, optional

1 crushed bud of garlic
salt as needed
$1^1/_3$ c. tomato puree

Simmer the onion in a little water. Add remaining ingredients and pour into the garbanzos. Cook slowly for 30 to 60 minutes. Yield: 4–6 servings.

Crock Pot Beans

1 lb. beans, dry
5 c. tomatoes, canned
2 T. molasses, optional

1 t. salt
1 t. garlic **or** onion powder
2 T. lemon juice

Soak beans in tomatoes for one hour in cold pot. Turn pot on and cook for 9–10 hours or overnight.

Puree of Kidney Beans, Lentils, Soybeans

4 c. cooked dry beans **or** canned
    kidney beans

$^1/_2$ c. water **or** gravy
1 large onion, chopped

Mash beans through a sieve, or place with the gravy (may use more than $^1/_2$ cup) in blender and blend until smooth. Add the chopped onion. Salt to taste. Pile into a casserole and heat through before serving. Consistency should resemble mashed potatoes. Serves 4–6.

Mashed Split Peas

1$\frac{1}{2}$ c. dried split peas
$\frac{1}{2}$ c. diced carrots
1 c. chopped onions

salt to taste
2 T. **Nut Cream or** water

Wash the peas and soak 2 hours. Do not drain, but add enough water to cover $\frac{1}{2}$". Add the carrots, onions, and salt. Cook the peas about 45–60 minutes to a mush adding water if necessary. Add the cream, blend well, using enough to give the consistency of mashed potatoes. Season. A few sautéed or raw onions may be added. Dilute leftover portions with water and use as gravy. Yield: 4–5 servings.

Lima Bean and Tomato Casserole

1 lb. dry lima beans
2 c. tomatoes
$\frac{1}{2}$ c. diced celery

2 sliced onions
2 t. sugar, optional
salt to taste

Soak the washed beans overnight and boil them in the water they soaked in until tender or nearly done. Add remaining ingredients and place in a casserole. Add more water if necessary and bake slowly 1 hour at 350°.

Frijoles Con Chili

3 onions, chopped
3 buds garlic, chopped
1 small can sliced pimientos **or** 1–2 bell
peppers, chopped

2 t. salt
1 c. broth **or** hot water
1 T. whole grain flour
4 c. cooked frijoles (any bean)

Simmer together for half an hour. Serve in soup bowls or over rice or grits. Serves 6.

Bean Pot

2 c. dry beans
1 large onion, chopped

salt

Wash and sort beans and soak 2–10 hours, covered 1" with water. Add more water to keep beans covered. Cook in a kettle with tight cover for 2–4 hours, or pressure at 5 pounds for 1 hour. Beans should be tender with some breaking up. The liquid will become quite thick when the beans are done. Makes about 5 cups.

Bold Print indicates items listed in the INDEX

V. ENTREES AND NUT MAIN DISHES

Lentil Pot

2 c. lentils
1 c. chopped onions
1 T. lemon juice, optional

1 c. tomatoes **or** chopped green
    pepper, optional
1 bay leaf
salt as needed

Wash and sort lentils, soak 1–2 hours, boil in water that covers lentils. Add remaining items after $1/2$ hour and cook about 20 to 30 minutes more. Salt and serve in soup bowls, or over rice or potatoes. Makes about $3^1/2$ cups.

Lentil Patties

2 c. lentils, well cooked
3 c. finely ground bread crumbs
1 onion, chopped

1 t. salt
1 c. water or more
2 T. chopped parsley

Mix ingredients. Form into patties. Place on floured cookie sheet. Bake at 350° for 20 to 30 minutes or until nicely browned. Makes 10–15 patties.

Baked Lentils

3 c. lentils
$1/4$ c. onions
2 t. salt

$1/2$ c. bread crumbs
2 c. tomatoes

Wash the lentils and soak in cold water 2 or more hours. Do not drain. Add the onions and boil 1 hour or until tender. Add salt when half done. Whirl tomatoes in blender and heat to the boiling point. Add to lentils which should be boiled sufficiently dry so that draining is not necessary. Place them in baking dish. Cover with bread crumbs, and bake in the oven until crumbs are a golden brown. Serves 6.

Bold Print indicates items listed in the INDEX

Tostado Filling

2 onions, chopped
1 t. garlic powder
2 c. tomatoes

2 t. salt, more or less
8 c. cooked beans

Cook first four ingredients until nearly done. Add beans and simmer 15 minutes. Blend to make paste. Pile in casserole serving dish and keep hot in oven. Serve over tostados or **Croutons** and top with chopped lettuce and tomatoes. Serves 8–12.

Soaked Soybeans

$3^1/_2$ c. dry soybeans

Place beans in a two-quart jar with enough cold water to fill the jar. Put top on jar and keep in refrigerator until needed for use in **Corn Bread** recipes, **Scalloped Potatoes**, **Soy Soufflé**, etc.

Chili Beans

4 c. cooked beans, red, soy, etc.
1 c. onion, chopped
$2^1/_2$ c. tomatoes

1 c. bell pepper, chopped
2 t. celery salt **or** other seasoning salt

Simmer slowly about 45 minutes. Good with rice or burgers, or serve in a soup bowl with a dollop of **Wheatonnaise**. Serves 4–6.

Soynuts I

1 c. soybeans

2 c. water

Soak beans for 48 hours and boil for 1 hour. Drain, sprinkle lightly with salt and spread out in a shallow pan. Roast at 350° for 45 minutes until crisp.

Bold Print indicates items listed in the INDEX

V. ENTREES AND NUT MAIN DISHES

Soynuts II

1 c. soybeans   3 c. boiling water

Boil for 30 minutes without prior soaking. Drain. Cover with water, add 1 teaspoon salt. Pressure cook at 10 pounds for 1 hour. Drain. Spread in flat pan and roast at 350° for 30 to 40 minutes, stirring if needed, until entirely dry and crisp.

Soy Patties I

2 c. mashed soybeans; **Garbanzos or**   ½ c. dry bread crumbs
other beans may be used   salt and sage if desired

Mix, shape into small balls. Roll in bread crumbs, flatten into patties and place on floured cookie tin. Bake at 350° for 20–30 minutes, until brown. Serves about 6.

Soy Patties II

1½ c. **Soaked Soybeans**   2 c. whole grain flour
1½ c. water   ¾ t. salt
2 T. flax seed **or** oatmeal

Grind first three ingredients in blender. Add flour, salt, and favorite seasonings such as onion powder, thyme, or ¼ teaspoon sage. Add 3 tablespoons flake yeast if desired. Spoon onto floured baking pan and flatten. Bake at 350° for about 45 minutes. Serves about 6.

Millet Patties

4 c. cooked **Millet**   2 t. onion powder
¼ c. **Nut Butter**   1 t. celery salt

Form into patties and brown in oven at 350° for about 35 minutes. Serves 6.

Bold Print indicates items listed in the INDEX

Sprouted Lentils

2 c. dry lentils
1 t. salt
$1^1/_4$ c. water

$^1/_2$ t. celery salt
$^1/_2$ c. onions

Sprout lentils by **Sprouting Instructions** for about 5 days. When sprouts are $^1/_2$" long they are ready for use. Put last four ingredients in blender and whirl to mix and grate onion fine. Add to lentils in a kettle and cook slowly for about 20 minutes, adding more water as it is needed to make broth. Serve with **Rice**, **Pasta**, or **Pizza**. Serves 4–6.

Soy Loaf

4 c. **Soaked Soybeans**
4 c. water
2 onions
1 c. raw rice **or** rolled oats

2 c. tomato puree
$1^1/_2$ t. salt
1 t. sage, scant
1 T. food yeast

Put the beans in blender with water and onions and grind until fine. Add to other ingredients. Pour into floured loaf pans or juice cans. Bake at 300° **or** steam for 3 hours. May pressure cook for 1 hour at 5 pounds. Serves 4–6. Serve with generous amounts of fresh parsley if desired.

Lentil-Nut Loaf

3 c. lentils, cooked
$^1/_2$ c. ground sunflower seed **or**
    chopped nuts
1 T. onion powder

$^1/_4$ t. sage
1 t. salt
$^1/_2$ c. rolled oats **or** bread crumbs
    (3 slices)

Mix well, using water to adjust consistency so that oats are quite wet. Bake in floured loaf pan for 1 hour at 350°. Serve with **Cashew Gravy**.

Hoppin' John

1 c. dry blackeyed peas
8 c. vegetable broth **or** water
1 c. uncooked rice

$1^1/_2$ t. salt or more
$^1/_2$ c. nuts

Wash and drain peas. Put peas and broth in a kettle. Boil 2 minutes. Remove from heat, cover, and let stand 1 hour. Add rice, nuts, and salt. Boil gently 1–2 hours until peas are almost tender. Do not stir after this time. Cover and boil gently about 60 minutes, until rice is tender. Makes 6 servings, 1 cup each.

Bold Print indicates items listed in the INDEX

LEGUMES

Soy Cheese Balls

2 c. **Soy Cottage Cheese or**
    chopped **Tofu**
2 c. cooked brown rice
2 green onions, finely chopped

$^1/_2$ t. salt, if needed
$^1/_2$ c. chopped parsley **or** green
    peppers

Shape into 2 dozen small balls, then roll in wheat germ. Bake at 375° for $^1/_2$ hour.

Chili Grits

1 small onion
$^1/_4$ green pepper
1 t. salt
1 t. mixed herbs

1 c. uncooked corn grits
1 c. cooked red beans
4 c. water

Place ingredients except beans in a kettle. Cook 1 hour, stirring occasionally. Add cooked beans, 1 or more cups. Makes 6 servings, about $^3/_4$ cup each.

Soy Soufflé

2 c. water
2 t. salt
2 T. minced onion
3 c. drained **Soaked Soybeans**

1 t. garlic powder
$^1/_4$ c. pimiento, chopped
1 t. mixed herbs

Liquefy beans in blender, adding 1 cup water to $1^1/_2$ cups beans. (This makes 4–5 cups pulp). Add other ingredients. Bake in floured pan $1^1/_2$ hours at 300°. This soufflé will not "fall." This may be served for breakfast on toast with a dressing.

Green Lima Beans with Fine Herbs

2 pkgs., 10 oz. each, frozen green lima
    beans, **or** about 1 qt. canned beans
1 t. lemon juice
1 T. chopped chives

1 T. minced parsley
1 t. tarragon
salt

Cook the lima beans in a little water until tender (about 30 to 45 minutes). Add all the seasonings. Serve as a main dish. Yield: 4–6 servings.

Bold Print indicates items listed in the INDEX

Greens Roast

2 parts greens, seasoned, cooked **or** parboiled
1 part beans, soaked overnight

salt as needed
1 part bread crumbs

Liquefy the greens in blender. Liquefy the beans in an equal quantity of broth or water. Add 1 teaspoon salt for each quart of liquefied beans. Add bread crumbs. Bake at 350° about 1 hour, until brown. Split peas also good in this recipe instead of beans. This roast has a very good biologic value. Serve with a **French Dressing** or favorite sour sauce.

Hommus Tahini

2 c. **Cooked Garbanzos or** green soybeans
$1/2$ c. sesame seed
1 clove garlic, optional

salt, if needed
1 T. chopped parsley, optional
3 T. lemon juice

Liquefy beans, salt (about $1/2$ teaspoon if **Garbanzos** are unsalted), garlic, and seed with barely enough bean broth to make blender turn. Sprinkle with garlic powder if clove garlic omitted. Serve over **Melba Toast** with parsley. Yield: 3–4 servings.

Baked Beans

6 c. any cooked legume
$1/2$ c. **Tomato Sauce or** 1 c. tomatoes
1 c. water
1 T. lemon juice

1 onion, chopped **or** left whole placed in center of pot
1 small clove garlic, chopped
salt to taste
1 T. molasses

Mix and place in a bean pot or baking dish. Bake at 350° for 1 hour or longer. Yield: 6–10 servings.

Creole

$1^1/4$ c. diced onion
2 tomatoes, peeled and diced, **or** 2 c. canned tomatoes
2 t. salt
1 bay leaf

$1/2$ c. **Tomato Sauce**
3 c. **Cooked Garbanzos**
$1/2$ c. hot water
hot **Brown Rice**

Sauté onion in water in a large skillet over low heat until tender. Add tomatoes, bay leaf and **Tomato Sauce**. Cover and simmer 15 minutes. Add **Garbanzos**. Cover and simmer 10 minutes longer. Serve in soup bowls over **Brown Rice**. Makes 6 servings.

Bold Print indicates items listed in the INDEX

LEGUMES

___

Paella-Garbanzos
(pie-el-ya)

6 c. vegetable broth
1 onion, chopped
1 clove garlic, minced
4–6 c. **Cooked Garbanzos**

3 ripe tomatoes, peeled and diced
or 3 c. canned tomatoes
2 c. brown rice, uncooked
2 t. salt

In a large kettle sauté the onion and garlic in a little water until tender. Add tomatoes and rice. Cook for 10 minutes, stirring frequently. Add salt and broth. Boil for $1^1/_4$ hours. Pour into baking dish. Add **Garbanzos**. Cover with a tight lid or foil. Place in a 350° oven and bake for 25 minutes. Serves 8–10.

"Salmon Loaf"

1 c. tomato juice
1 c. water

1 c. soy flour
$1^1/_2$ t. onion salt

Whirl in blender until smooth and pour into floured baking dish. Bake at 400° about 40 minutes until tan crust forms. Cool and turn onto a platter. Serve hot or cold as main dish with a sauce. Use sliced with **Wheatonnaise** for sandwiches. It is expected that loaves made with soy flour will fall slightly. Do not be disappointed. The flavor is not altered, and the "falling" develops a cheese-like consistency.

Blackeyed Peas, East Indian Style

3 c. water
1 c. dry blackeyed peas
1 onion, chopped
1 t. honey

2 T. coconut, grated **or** shredded
$^1/_4$ t. paprika
salt to taste

Soak peas in water 2 hours or overnight. Boil in soaking water until tender. Add remaining ingredients and cook 10 to 20 minutes longer to blend flavors. Yield: 3–4 servings.

Blackeyed Pea Loaf

2 c. blackeyed peas, cooked
2 c. water
1 large onion
2 t. mixed herbs as desired

$^1/_3$ c. rolled oats
$1^1/_2$ c. corn meal
salt to taste

Blend first 5 ingredients in blender. Pour into corn meal. Bake in a loaf pan at 350° for $1–1^1/_2$ hours. The darker brown it gets the more firm the slices become, to the point that the slices may be used as Corn Bread. Serve hot or cold with a rich gravy.

Holiday Roast

2 c. water
1 1/2 c. rolled oats
3 c. cooked rice
3 c. cooked grits
1 c. bread crumbs, add last

1/2–1 c. chopped nuts
1 c. chopped onions or 1/2 T. onion
   powder
3/4 t. ground sage

Mix and bake in a floured baking dish about 1–2 hours at 350°. Serve with **Holiday Gravy**. Serves about 12. Salt to taste.

Carrot Roast

4 c. grated carrots
4 c. cooked **Rice or Garbanzos**
1 c. bread crumbs
1/2 c. water

1/2 c. onion
thyme
salt

Mix ingredients. Bake 1 hour at 350°. Serve with **Gravy**. Yield: 4 servings.

Bread Dressing

15 slices bread, cubed
3 c. water
2 onions
1 T. Vegex

1/2 t. sage
1/3 c. **Soy Base**
1/8 t. salt
1/2 t. garlic powder

Whirl all ingredients except bread in the blender. The onions may be left in chips if desired. Mix the bread and place in floured baking dish. Bake at 350° for 1 hour. Serves 6.

Corn Pudding

1/2 c. **soaked soybeans**
1 1/2 c. fresh or frozen corn
1/2 c. water or vegetable stock
1 t. salt

1/4 t. basil
1 c. whole kernel corn
2 T. chopped parsley

Blend smooth the first 5 ingredients. Add the last two. Pour into oiled baking pan. Bake at 450° for 10 minutes, then at 350° 1 1/4 hours, uncovered.

Bold Print indicates items listed in the INDEX

V. ENTREES AND NUT MAIN DISHES

GRAINS
_____

Macaroni or Noodles with Green Peppers and Onions

1½ recipes of **Macaroni or Noodles**   salt
2 buds garlic   2 large green peppers
¼ c. water   3 large onions

Cut the peppers and onions very fine, mash the garlic in an iron skillet, and sauté them all lightly in the water. Cook **Macaroni** until tender in salted, boiling water, drain and mix with the vegetables. Pour into a hot serving dish and sprinkle with bread crumbs or nut crumbs. Bake 10 minutes at 400°. Sliced black olives may be added if desired. Serves 6.

Noodles with Fresh Asparagus

1 recipe **Noodles** (8 oz.)   salt
2 lbs. asparagus   crumbs
¼ c. water   2 buds garlic, crushed

Cook the **Noodles** in boiling, salted water and drain. Cook the asparagus until tender and drain. Sauté the crushed garlic in the water 2 minutes, then add the **Noodles** and mix well with a little salt. Pour into a hot serving dish and make a bed for the asparagus. Lay hot asparagus on the **Noodles** and sprinkle liberally with crumbs. Serves 5 or 6.

Baked Macaroni and Olives

1 c. uncooked **Macaroni**   2 c. water in which the **Macaroni**
½ c. chopped ripe olives   was cooked
2 T. chopped onion   ¼ c. flour
¼ c. **Tomato Paste**   salt **and** celery to taste

Drop **Macaroni** into boiling, salted water, and cook until it is well done. **Dextrinize** the flour in a small pan. Add remaining ingredients to make gravy. Have the **Macaroni** well drained; and while it is hot, put it into the gravy. Turn into a baking dish. Sprinkle bread crumbs over the top and press down so they become moistened through. Bake at 350° for 30–45 minutes. Serves 4.

Bold Print indicates items listed in the INDEX

Corn with Spaghetti

1 recipe **Spaghetti or Noodles**
2 c. fresh **or** canned corn
1 green pepper, chopped

1 t. salt
2 onions, chopped

Cook the **Spaghetti** or **Noodles** (substitute if desired 8 ounces of commercial soy spaghetti) in boiling, salted water and drain them. Sauté the onions and green pepper in water until tender. Mix, season, and pour into a casserole dish. Top with small **Croutons**. Bake 1 hour at 350°. Serves 4.

Baked Macaroni and Lentils

$^3/_4$ c. lentils
1 recipe of **Macaroni**
1 big onion, chopped

$^1/_2$ c. **Tomato Sauce**
$^1/_2$ green pepper, chopped
crumbs

Soak lentils 2 or more hours, cover $^1/_2$″ with water and cook them 1–2 hours. Add lentils to the drained **Macaroni** which has cooked in boiling, salted water (substitute 8 ounces of commercial wheat macaroni). Sauté the onion and green pepper in a little water until soft and mix with **Macaroni**. Pour into a floured baking dish. Cover with a mixture of fine crumbs. Bake at 350° for 25 minutes. Serves 4.

Chinese Pepper Steak

2 c. **Gluten**
$^1/_4$ c. water
1 t. salt or more
$^1/_4$ c. toasted sesame seed

4 c. sliced celery, tomatoes, green peppers, and onions mixed (select any 2 of these 4)
1–2 t. **Chicken Style Seasoning**

Cut **Gluten** in thin strips. Sauté the vegetables and seasonings in skillet, mixing gently but thoroughly. Cook until just tender. Add **Gluten**. Serve over **Rice**, **Grits**, or **Millet**. Serves 6.

Bold Print indicates items listed in the INDEX

GRAINS

Spaghetti and Burger Balls

SAUCE

$^1/_4$ c. water
1$^1/_2$ c. chopped onion
$^1/_2$ c. chopped green pepper
1$^1/_2$ t. salt
1 t. sweet basil

1 t. garlic powder, optional
1 c. vegetable broth or water as needed
4$^1/_2$ c. **Tomato Paste** or **Sauce**

Put first four ingredients in pan and sauté until onion is clear. Add the remaining ingredients. Simmer 30 minutes.

BALLS

1 c. oats
$^1/_2$ c. whole grain flour or more
1 onion, chopped
$^1/_4$ c. water
$^1/_4$ t. sage, optional

$^1/_2$ c. chopped almonds
2 c. water
$^1/_4$ t. salt
3–4 c. chopped **Gluten** (substitute 3 c. mashed **Garbanzos**)

Coarsely grind dry oats in blender. **Dextrinize** oats and flour. Sauté onion in $^1/_4$ cup water. Mix all ingredients and shape 1–2″ balls. Bake on floured cookie sheet about 30 minutes at 350°. (This recipe also makes good roast or patties.) Mix sauce and balls and pour over hot **Spaghetti** or **Macaroni**. Yield: 30 to 40 balls, 6 cups sauce. Serves 6.

Spaghetti and Chee Sauce

1 c. **Garbanzos**
1$^1/_4$ c. water
2–4 T. lemon juice, as desired
$^1/_4$ c. yeast flakes

1$^1/_2$ t. salt
1 t. onion powder
1 c. tomatoes

Blend the above ingredients in blender, pour into cooked **Soy** or **Whole Wheat Macaroni**. To cook the pasta, place 1 pound of **Soy**, **Whole Wheat**, or buckwheat spaghetti in 3 quarts of boiling water with 1 tablespoon salt. Boil about 15 to 20 minutes. Drain. After mixing with the **Chee Sauce**, bake 1 hour at 350°. Serves about 6. Variation: Leave the **Garbanzos** whole and leave out the 1$^1/_4$ cups water. Top with seasoned bread crumbs or chopped nuts.

Bold Print indicates items listed in the INDEX

Lasagne

4 c. canned tomatoes, drained
1 large onion, sliced fine
1 T. honey
1 t. salt or more

2 T. sweet basil
1 clove garlic
8 oz. **Lasagne Noodles**, cooked

Mix ingredients except the **Noodles** and simmer until onions are cooked. Spread a layer of the sauce on the bottom of pyrex pan. Lay on strips of cooked **Lasagne Noodles** side by side. Cover generously with **Tofu** cubes or crumbs. Repeat the layers, ending with the sauce. May sprinkle with bread crumbs if desired. Bake at 375° for 1 hour. Variations: Substitute any cooked beans or peas for **Tofu**. Serve the sauce separately from the **Lasagne Noodles** without baking. Use the sauce on **Pizza**. Serves about 4 or 5.

Macaroni Chee with Peanuts

1 recipe **Macaroni**
$^3/_4$ c. chopped toasted peanuts
1 c. **Golden Sauce**
$^3/_4$ c. fine crumbs

$1^1/_2$ c. water
1 t. salt
2 T. flour

Cook **Macaroni** (or **Spaghetti**) in boiling, salted water until tender. Drain off water. Stir in the other ingredients except peanuts and crumbs. Cook slowly until thickened, stirring constantly. Add about half of both the crumbs and the peanuts. Pour into ungreased baking dish. Sprinkle with remaining crumbs and peanuts. Brown at 375° about 30 minutes. Makes 4 servings.

Nuttose

1 c. tomato pulp
$^2/_3$ c. warm water
$^2/_3$ c. whole grain flour
$^1/_3$ c. starch

1 t. salt
$^1/_4$ c. **Nut Butter**
$^1/_4$ t. each of sage **and** marjoram

Put the water, seasonings, and **Nut Butter** in the blender and whirl. Add the tomato, flour, and starch, whirling until smooth. Pour into a floured tube cake pan or large juice can. Steam for 2–3 hours in a **Covered Steamer**. Unmold. Cool uncovered for several hours. Slice for sandwiches or cut in wedges, garnish with parsley, and serve as main dish. Yield: 4–6 servings.

Bold Print indicates items listed in the INDEX

GRAINS

Gluten

8 c. wheat flour (white **or** whole wheat)   3 c. water

Mix, knead well, place ball of dough in large mixing bowl and cover with water. Allow to soften for $\frac{1}{2}$ hour or overnight. Remove the starch from the ball by kneading and working it in the large bowl of water, keeping the dough together. Pour off the first two washings into a storage container to allow the starch to settle. The fluid part is high in B-vitamins, iron, and other nutrients and should be used in cooking or baking.

Continue working the ball of dough in water, pouring off the water and adding new until no more white cloud of starch appears in the water. The tough, elastic lump is mainly gluten, the protein of wheat.

8 c. water   2 t. salt (seasoning salt may
                                         be preferred)

Bring to a rolling boil in a very large kettle. Trim slices from the gluten lump with kitchen shears or scissors. The shape of each portion trimmed off will be determined by whether choplets, scallops, stew beef, or other styles are desired. Cut the pieces a little smaller than finished product is expected as gluten swells as it cooks. Let the pieces fall to the bottom of the boiling liquid. As they rise to the top they will be set and firm and will not stick together as readily as when first dropped in. Boil gently about 30 to 35 minutes uncovered. At this point the gluten may be canned, frozen or prepared in roasts, stews, gravies, or ground and used as ground beef is used in burgers or loaves.

Millet Loaf

1 onion, chopped
1 c. celery, chopped
2 c. **Gluten or** $\frac{1}{2}$ c. sunflower seed
$\frac{1}{4}$ c. water
$\frac{3}{4}$ c. uncooked millet

2 c. "**Mushroom**" Soup
2 c. water
$\frac{1}{8}$ t. sage **or** thyme
garlic salt
$\frac{1}{2}$ c. chopped olives

Sauté first three ingredients in $\frac{1}{4}$ cup water. Add remaining ingredients. Pour into a loaf pan and bake $1\frac{1}{2}$ hours at 325°. Variation: use rice in place of millet. Any kind of nuts may be substituted for sunflower seed. Serves 6.

Bold Print indicates items listed in the INDEX

Pizza

PIZZA CRUST

Use **Whole Wheat Bread** recipe or **Pie Crust** for pizza crust. Take the dough for one bread recipe and divide into 2 or 3 portions. Roll each portion out on a floured surface to about 13″ in diameter. Shape on bottom and sides of a 12″ pizza pan. Cover lightly and let rise in warm place approximately 20 minutes until light. Prick with a fork. Bake in preheated 350° oven until barely turning brown (about 12 minutes). Remove and cool.

SAUCE

$^1/_2$ c. water
$^1/_4$ c. bell pepper
1 c. tomato puree
1 c. canned tomatoes
1 t. honey

1 c. onion, chopped
1 c. ground **Gluten or Garbanzos**
3 cloves garlic, minced
1 t. mixed herbs

Sauté onion, bell pepper, and garlic in water. Add remaining ingredients and simmer 10 minutes to blend flavors. Add about $^1/_2$ teaspoon salt or season to taste.

Spread sauce over two baked **Pizza Crusts**. Drizzle **Chee Sauce**, or dot **Agar Cheese**, or sprinkle **Soy Cheese** squares or crumbs over top. May use chopped olives, sauteed onions or eggplant, nuts, soybeans, or any article desired. Keep the number of articles used to about three, to avoid a complex mixture. Serve with tomato wedges. Sprinkle with diluted lemon juice. Serves 6.

Gluten and Pasta
Macaroni or Spaghetti

3 c. **Gluten**, cut small
1 c. tomato juice
1 T. yeast flakes
1 T. flour

1 medium onion, chopped
1 recipe of **Macaroni**
salt and mixed herbs

Cook the **Macaroni** into boiling water. Place onion in a large kettle and sauté in a little water until tender. Add first four ingredients and bring to a boil. Add salt and herbs to season. Pour over the **Macaroni** in a floured dish. Bake at 350° for 30 minutes. Serves 6.

Bold Print indicates items listed in the INDEX

GRAINS
___

"Arroz con Pollo"

2 c. **Cooked Garbanzos**   2 c. canned tomatoes
4 c. water   2 t. salt
1 t. basil   2 c. brown rice, raw
4 onions, sliced

Mix all ingredients in 3 quart casserole. Cover and bake at 325° for 2–3 hours, adding more water or tomato juice if necessary. Serve with tossed salad or cucumber. NOTE: May be cooked in pot on stove if preferred. Do not stir after first 20 minutes as rice becomes sticky. Serves 6–10.

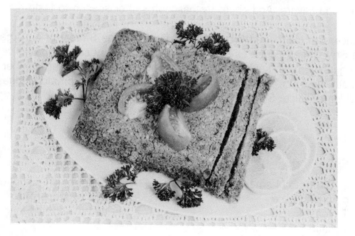

Holiday Roast, page 91

Bold Print indicates items listed in the INDEX

Chow Mein

1 c. onions, chopped
1 c. celery, chopped
1 c. sliced olives, **Gluten, or Garbanzos**

1 T. starch
1 t. salt, more or less
1–2 c. "**Mushroom**" **Soup**

Mix the last three ingredients in a saucepan and bring to a boil, stirring constantly. Add other ingredients and simmer for 15 minutes. Serve over **Dry Rice**, **Macaroni**, **Millet**, or **Corn Grits**. For variety, add 2–4 cups of beans or **Sprouts**, 1 cup of chopped bell pepper.

Split Peas and Rice Casserole

3 c. split peas, cooked
2 c. cooked **Dry Rice**
2 c. canned tomatoes

1/2 c. onion, chopped fine
1/2 c. **Tomato Paste**, optional
salt to taste

In a floured baking dish make layers of peas, tomatoes, and onion. Sprinkle with salt if needed. Cover with **Tomato Paste** if desired. Bake at 400° for 20 minutes. Serve with **Tomato Gravy**. Serves 6.

Split Pea Casserole

1 small onion
1/4 c. water
2 T. soy flour
2 1/4 c. water

2 1/2 c. cooked split peas
1 c. uncooked, rolled oats
1 c. cooked beans **or** 1/2 c. pecans
1/2 t. salt

Chop onion and cook in 1/4 cup water until tender. Beat the soy flour and water in a large bowl. Stir onion and rest of ingredients into soy flour mixture. Pour into floured baking pan. Bake at 350° about 50 minutes. Makes 4 servings.

Chop Suey

1/4 c. water
1 onion, chopped
1 c. celery, chopped
1 c. **Cooked Garbanzos**
1/2 c. water

4 c. **Sprouts (Mung Beans** best, but try any kind)
1/4 c. toasted chopped almonds, optional
1 T. **Chicken Style Seasoning**

Cook first three ingredients until tender. Add **Sprouts** and water and cook until almost tender. Add **Garbanzos**. Serve over **Rice** or **Noodles**. Top with ground, toasted almonds. Serves 3–4.

Bold Print indicates items listed in the INDEX

Potato Entrees

(See VEGETABLE section for many casseroles using potatoes, all of which are suitable for entrees. In the VEGETABLE section are many dishes using corn, eggplant, carrots, squash, turnips, sweet potatoes, and others, which are good entrees.)

Lima Bean Casserole

1$^1/_4$ c. dry limas	1$^1/_2$ c. water
4 c. water	1 c. bread crumbs
$^1/_2$ small onion	1$^1/_4$ t. salt **or** to taste
$^1/_4$ c. soy flour	

Soak beans in 4 cups water overnight. Adjust water level until beans are covered with about $^1/_2$" of water. Cook until tender or pressure cook. Put the flour in skillet and heat while stirring until nutty odor is produced. Cool slightly. Add water and salt. Cook until thickened. Pour into beans with $^1/_2$ cup bread crumbs. Pour into a casserole. Top with other half of bread crumbs, and bake at 350° about 30 minutes. Serves 4.

Pecan Loaf

1 c. pecan or cashew meal	4 c. soft bread crumbs
$^1/_2$ c. sunflower seed	1$^1/_2$ t. salt
2 c. cooked rice	1 t. sweet basil

Whiz in blender and add to above:

1$^1/_2$ c. water	$^2/_3$ c. soy or whole wheat flour
1 onion	

Mix the first 6 items in a bowl. Blend the last 3 items and combine with the first. Pour into a well oiled loaf pan. Bake at 375° for 1$^1/_2$ hours. May substitute 1 cup of whole kernel corn in the recipe for the nuts and seeds if needed to conserve calories. Serves 6–8.

Peanut Meat

1$^1/_2$ c. toasted peanuts	2 t. salt
3 c. water	$^1/_3$ c. soy flour
$^1/_2$ c. cornstarch	

Blend all ingredients together. Bake covered for 1$^1/_2$ hours at 300°. Slice when cold. Serve on sandwiches. Good cubed and mixed with rice and Almond Gravy.

Bold Print indicates items listed in the INDEX

Cashew Casserole

1 c. celery, chopped
1 c. onion, chopped
1/4 c. olives, chopped
1/4 c. water
1/2 c. cashews

2 c. **Cooked Garbanzos**
2 c. rolled oats
1 t. salt or more
2 c. water

Sauté first four ingredients lightly. Whirl **Garbanzos** in blender with enough water or broth to turn blender easily. Mix all ingredients. Bake in a floured casserole at 350° for about 1 hour. Serves 4.

Corn Tamale Pie

1 c. corn meal
2 1/2 c. water
2 c. whole kernel corn
3/4 c. chopped olives
1/2 c. **Tomato Sauce or** 3 c. canned tomatoes, omitting the 2 1/2 c. water

1 c. chopped onion
1 t. salt or **Chicken Style Seasoning**
1 c. chopped green peppers, optional

Make **Corn Meal Mush** of corn meal, water (or juice from draining the tomatoes) and salt. Simmer remaining ingredients until onion is beginning to be transparent. Combine all ingredients. Pour into a baking dish. Bake at 350° for 1 hour. Serves 4.

Scalloped Eggplant

8 c. steamed eggplant cubes
2 c. bread crumbs
1/2 t. salt or more

1/2 c. **Soy Base, Double Strength Soy Milk, or Basic Cream Sauce**, medium

Mix and bake in a casserole dish topped with bread crumbs. Bake at 350° for 45 minutes.

Shepherd Pie

2 c. cooked peas **or** beans
2 c. sautéed onions
2 c. diced, cooked carrots

2 c. Irish potato chunks, cooked and chopped in jackets
2 c. **Holiday Gravy**
Mashed Potatoes for icing

Place all vegetables together in a deep casserole dish. Pour **Gravy** over vegetables to fill about 1/3 of the dish. Spread **Mashed Potatoes** on top as an icing, or use **Pie Crust** as a topping. Heat in oven for about 30 minutes before serving. Lightly brown the icing peaks. If **Pie Crust** is used, bake at 350° for 30 to 50 minutes. Serve as a single dish with spring onions and carrot strips. Serves 4–6.

BURGERS AND PATTIES
___

Serving Suggestions for Burgers and Patties

1. With **Bread** and **Spreads** as a sandwich.
2. Eaten from the hand as bread when baked crisp.
3. Used as a base for piled-on vegetables or **Gravies** in **Open Face Sandwich**.
4. Stacked irregularly in a casserole, covered with **Gravy** or **Sauce** and baked until set.

Pea Patties

4 c. crowder **or Blackeyed Peas** $1/2$ c. brown flour (wheat **or** rye)

Cook peas or use leftovers. Place peas in blender with enough broth or water to blend easily. Add flour, more or less, to make a thick paste. Salt if necessary. Dip by scoopfuls and flatten onto a cookie tin. Bake at 300° for $1 1/2$ hours. Makes 24 small patties. Serve at breakfast instead of toast, or at dinner under **Spanish Rice**.

Buckwheat Crispies

$1/2$ c. **Buckwheat Groats**   1 large onion, chopped
1 c. boiling water   1 c. flour, approximate
$1/4$ t. salt   1 c. water, approximate

Dextrinize groats for 5 minutes, stirring constantly. Add salt, onions, and boiling water, cover, and cook gently 10 minutes. Add enough whole wheat or buckwheat flour and water to make a dough the consistency needed to make either round balls from a stiff dough; or flat patties from a thinner batter. Bake at 350°, 20–25 minutes until crusty brown. Serve with **Holiday Gravy**.

Split Pea Patties

$2 1/2$ c. cooked split peas $1/3$ c. water
$1/2$ small onion $1/2$ t. salt
1 c. fine, dry bread crumbs $1/4$ c. whole grain flour
$1/4$ c. chopped nuts or seeds, optional $1/4$ c. shredded carrots, optional

Mash split peas with a fork. Chop onion finely. Mix all ingredients. Shape into 12 patties. Bake at 350° until browned on both sides. Makes 6 servings, 2 patties each. Serve with **Rice Cream**.

Bold Print indicates items listed in the INDEX

Okra Patties

4 c. cooked okra
whole grain flour

salt
onion **or** garlic powder

Add enough flour to make a thick paste with the okra. With a potato masher puree the okra mixture until it is as smooth as possible. Add salt and seasoning. Form into patties and bake on floured cookie tin at 350° about 45 minutes until brown crust forms. Serve with dinner vegetables, or with **Mustard** and **Catsup** as a burger.

Eggplant Patties

2 medium eggplants
1 T. onion powder
$^1/_2$ c. rye, barley, **or** whole wheat flour

water **or** vegetable broth
salt

Steam whole eggplant in small amount of water. Chop small enough for blender to handle. Use just enough water or broth to blend eggplant, skin and all. Pour up and add flour, onion powder, and enough bread crumbs or **Breading Meal** to make a stiff batter. If desired add $^1/_4$ cup finely chopped nuts for each 4 cups of batter. Salt to taste. Shape patties, place on floured baking sheet, bake at 350° for $^1/_2$ hour. Serve with **Catsup** or **Mustard**. Yield: 10 to 12 patties.

Oat Burgers or Loaf

2 c. cooked oatmeal
1 raw potato
$^1/_2$ c. onion
$^1/_4$ c. walnuts **or** other nuts, optional

1–2 c. bread crumbs
1 t. salt
$^1/_2$ t. sage

Grind potato, onion, and a little water in blender if needed. Mix with cooked oatmeal. Add remaining items and mix. Use more crumbs if water used in blender. Form patties or make into roast. Bake in tin at 350° until nicely browned. Burgers require 45 minutes, turning after 30 minutes. Loaf requires about 60 minutes. Serves 4.

Pecan Patties

2 medium potatoes
1 medium onion
1 t. salt
1 c. water

$^1/_2$ c. whole grain flour
$^1/_2$ c. ground pecans
1 c. bread crumbs

Place first four ingredients in blender and chop finely. Mix with remaining ingredients. Shape into patties and bake 45 minutes at 350° on baking sheet. Turn at 30 minutes. Variation: may be used as a roast. Bake for 1 hour at 350° in a floured baking dish. Serves 4.

V. ENTREES AND NUT MAIN DISHES

<u>STEWS, SOUPS, AND CHOWDERS</u>

Soups should be hearty, having a large proportion of solid food in relation to the liquid portion, as too much liquid interferes with digestion. All liquid drained from vegetables, **Pastas**, or other foods should be saved in a special jar in the refrigerator to use in soups and stews as well as in the preparation of breads and vegetarian entrees instead of water.

I urge everyone to invest in an electric blender. In a few seconds one can make purees and sauces. Small bits of left over vegetables can be whirled in a little stock to thicken soups.

Care must be used in making soups to keep them simple. It is not healthful to throw together a large number of different types of vegetables. To do so places a burden on the digestive organs. Two, or at most three, different vegetables in a stew, which will be served with a simple salad such as sliced cucumber or lettuce wedges, can be better accepted.

Soups are especially welcome in cold weather. When served with **Dry Rice**, **Croutons**, or **Melba Toast** in generous quantities they may form the entire meal. If thickening is desired, try to use for this purpose some of the flours not used so frequently in breads, such as buckwheat, barley, millet, rye, etc. In this way the trace elements carried in these grains can also be made available to the body. Do not forget that small portions of break-fast cereals, corn bread crusts and crumbs, or tiny bits of leftover legumes can be whirled in the blender with some of the vegetable stock to thicken soups. Dumplings should be used often to thicken soups.

Blending of the flavors in soups requires long, slow cooking. The herbs permeate the solid portions. Experiment with many different herbs and seasonings. Garnish soup bowls according to the following suggestions:

Garnish Suggestions for Soups

Almonds, chopped and toasted
Avocado, balls or slices
Cereals, whole wheat, **Granola** or **Maranola**
Cream, **Soy Sour**
Croutons made in different shapes
Chives, chopped
Cucumber, thin slices or chopped
Dill, chopped and fresh
Green pepper, chopped
Lemon or lime slices

Nuts, chopped and roasted
Olives, chopped ripe
Orange rind, grated
Parsley, tiny sprigs **or** chopped
Pimiento Cream
Popcorn, ground or whole
Radish slices
Scallion slices
Seed powder
Watercress, minced

Bold Print indicates items listed in the INDEX

Potato Soup

4 large potatoes
2 large onions
2 c. water
1 t. salt

1 T. whole grain flour
2 c. rich **Soy Milk or Basic Cream Sauce**

Cut potatoes and onions in small pieces. Mix remaining ingredients (except **Soy Milk**) in a blender and add to potatoes and onions. Cook slowly, stirring occasionally. When vegetables are tender add **Soy Milk**. Reheat but do not boil. Serves 4. Variation: The addition of cooked barley and a tablespoon of chopped fresh mint gives a delightful flavor and texture to this soup.

Garbanzo Soup

Place in blender, 2 cups of **Cooked Garbanzos** with enough water or **Soy Milk** to bring to the consistency of soup. Add onion if desired. Yield: 4 servings.

Soy Corn Chowder

3 c. green soybeans
1 c. water
1 c. chopped green onions
3 c. cream style corn
1 c. stewed tomatoes

1 t. salt
2 c. **Soy Milk or Basic Cream Sauce**
Sprinkle of herbs if desired

Cook beans and onions in 1 cup water. When tender add corn, tomatoes, and salt. Add rich **Soy Milk** when ready to serve. Dip over squares of **Corn Bread**. Yield 10 to 12 servings, 1 cup each.

Cream of "Mushroom" Soup

2 c. **Cooked Garbanzos**
1 c. minced celery
1/2 c. minced onion
1/4 c. water
2 T. whole grain flour
2 c. water

2 c. **Soy Milk or Basic Cream Sauce**, medium
1/2 t. salt
1/4 c. minced parsley
1–4 T. yeast flakes, to taste

Gently sauté the first five ingredients together until tender. Add remaining ingredients. Do not boil. Serve with **Spoon Bread**. Serves 4–6. Variations: Instead of garbanzos may use 1–3 cups whole kernel or creamed corn, dumplings or olives.

Certain species of mushrooms have been reported to be cancer-producing in animals. It would seem wise to omit mushrooms from the dietary. You will find this cream soup an acceptable substitute.

STEWS, SOUPS, AND CHOWDERS
___

Black Bean Soup

2 c. black beans
2 onions
2 carrots **or** stalks of celery

2 t. salt
2–3 qts. water
2 t. basil

Soak the beans overnight in cold water, drain and bring to a boil with 2–3 quarts cold water. Skim and add all the other ingredients. Cover very tightly and simmer for 4 hours, adding more water, if necessary. Strain through a sieve or whirl in blender with a little water. The soup should be like heavy cream. Add more salt if necessary. This delicious soup is even better the day after it is made. Serve hot with a lemon wedge as garnish. Serves 8. May use as a gravy over roasts, **Patties** or **Dry Rice**.

Mexican Bean Soup

2 c. pink beans **or** chick peas
2 minced onions
2 buds garlic

salt as needed
2 qts. water
$1/2$ c. **Tomato Sauce**

Soak the beans or peas overnight, drain and cover with 2 quarts lukewarm water. Mince the onions and garlic and add to beans or peas. Cover and gently cook 2 hours (**Garbanzos** will require 3 or more). Fifteen minutes before it is done, mix in the **Tomato Sauce**. May be pureed or the beans left whole in the soup. Also, try pureeing half the beans, giving the soup body. Serves 8.

Cucumber Soup
Serve Cold

3 c. cucumber chunks (about 3 large
  cucumbers)
2 T. water
3 c. broth **or** water
3 T. whole grain flour
$1/2$ c. chopped onion

1 c. **Soy Milk or Basic Cream Sauce**
salt as needed
1 T. minced parsley, optional
1 T. chopped green onion

Peel cucumbers and cook on low heat in 2 tablespoons water for 10 minutes. Add flour to cucumber, then add the broth. Heat **Soy Milk** to boiling point with parsley and onion and add to soup. If a creamy soup is desired, whirl in blender until smooth. Chill and serve with chopped green onion for garnish. Serves about 6.

Bold Print indicates items listed in the INDEX

Basic Cream Soup

Use 1½ or 2 cups of any canned or frozen vegetable. Use 1 cup thin **Basic Cream Sauce**. Liquefy vegetables or put through a coarse sieve, and add to the cream sauce. Season to taste and serve hot. Allow about 1 cup per serving.

Jacob's Lentil Stew

1 c. lentils
4 c. cold water
1 c. tiny white onions
1 clove garlic, chopped
3 carrots, sliced

(optional ingredients—use some or all)
2 t. salt
2 t. lemon juice
1 c. diced potato

Wash, then soak lentils overnight in 4 cups cold water. In the morning cook lentils ½ hour and then add all other ingredients. Cook until vegetables are tender. Serves 3–4.

Fresh English Pea Soup

4 c. shelled English peas
1 c. water

½ t. salt
2 T. whole grain flour **or** 1 T. starch

Liquefy the ingredients together in a blender. Bring to a boil while stirring constantly. Simmer for 3 minutes and serve. Serves 4.

Fresh Cream of Corn Soup

4 c. corn cut from cob
1½ c. **Soy or Nut Milk**

2 T. chopped green onions
1 t. salt

Place last two ingredients in a large sauce pan and heat together until onions are cooked. Liquefy corn and **Soy Milk** and add to cooked onions. Bring to a boil and serve with seasoned **Croutons** or **Melba Toast**. Serves 4.

Cream of Chestnut Soup

1 c. chestnuts
3–4 c. water

2 T. starch
1½ t. salt

Roast the chestnuts in the shell at 250° for 45 minutes. Shell chestnuts. Mix all ingredients and liquefy. Bring to a boil. Serve over **Croutons** or **Dry Rice**. Serves 4.

Bold Print indicates items listed in the INDEX

STEWS, SOUPS, AND CHOWDERS
_____

Chick Pea Soup

2 c. cooked chick peas (**Garbanzos**)
$1/4$ c. grated onion

$1/4$ c. pimiento
$1/2$ t. salt

Cook for 20 minutes to blend flavors. Add 1 cup **Soy Milk** or **Vegetarian Cream** at time of serving. Serve as a gravy if desired with **Corn Grits** or **Brown Rice**. Serves 4.

Split Pea Soup

6 c. water
$1/2$ c. rice
2 c. split peas
2 t. salt

1 c. chopped onions
$1/2$ c. diced carrots
$1/2$ c. celery, chopped
$1/2$ t. basil

Cook rice 1 hour in water. Add split peas and cook another hour. Add remaining ingredients and continue cooking about $1/2$ hour.

Ragout (ra-goo) of Vegetables

$2^1/2$ c. carrots
$2^1/2$ c. young turnips **or** potatoes
6 small onions
$1/4$ c. water

3 T. whole grain flour
a sprinkle of herbs
$2^1/2$ c. vegetable broth **or** water
salt to taste

Cut carrots in rounds and turnips in wedges. Braise carrots, turnips, and onions in a saucepan with $1/4$ cup water. Add the flour and continue cooking a few minutes. Add remaining ingredients. Let boil gently under cover until well done, and the gravy is reduced to a nice consistency. **Dumplings** go well with **Ragout**, or serve with **Rice** or **Croutons**. Serves 4.

Bean-Corn Soup

4 c. water
2 c. corn
2 cloves garlic

1 c. dry white beans
1 onion, quartered
salt to taste

Soak beans in water 2 or more hours. Cook everything together, except corn, until tender. Puree in blender, adding additional water or **Soy Milk** if needed. Add corn. Heat. Serves 4.

Bold Print indicates items listed in the INDEX

Cream of Cabbage Soup

1 c. vegetable broth
3 c. shredded cabbage
2 T. minced onion
1/2 t. thyme

1/2 t. salt
1 c. **Soy Milk or Basic Cream Sauce**
2 T. minced parsley

Cook first five ingredients for about 6 minutes. Stir in **Nut or Soy Milk**. Serve with **Croutons**. Serves 3–4.

Citron Melon Soup

8 c. cubed citron
2 T. water
1 t. herbs
2 T. whole grain flour

1 T. food yeast
salt to taste
1/2 c. **Nut Milk**

Put 2 tablespoons water more or less in a large kettle. Add the cubed melon and begin heating at very low flame. Citron is an easily stored melon that usually grows wild in gardens and fields and is not eaten because of its gourd-like flavor. This unpleasant flavor is banished with slow, long cooking. The melon stores a lot of water which is released on heating gently. After 1 hour of boiling time blend and add the last five ingredients. More flour may be needed for thickening. Serve with **Pulled Melba Toast** or **Maranola** for a delicious, unusual soup. Serves 6.

Lentil and Tomato Soup

2 c. mashed lentils
2 c. stewed tomatoes
boiling water, to make 6 c. total

1 c. **Steamed Rice**
1/2 t. onion salt
salt to taste

Rub lentils and tomatoes through sieve or put in blender. Add **Rice**, seasonings, and enough water to make 6 cups. Reheat and serve with **Croutons**. Serves 6, about 1 cup each.

Vichyssoise
hot or cold

4 bunches leeks, small or medium
4 c. thinly sliced potato
1 t. lemon juice, optional

salt and herb seasoning
1 qt. broth
2 c. **Soy or Nut Milk**

Chop only the white parts of the leeks (or spring onions). Put ingredients in pan. Simmer 20 minutes. Whirl in blender with **Nut or Soy Milk** and lemon juice. Add salt and seasoning. To serve hot, heat without boiling. Serves 6.

V. ENTREES AND NUT MAIN DISHES

STEWS, SOUPS, AND CHOWDERS

Split Pea Soup

4 c. water
2 c. dry split peas
1 sliced onion

(optional ingredients, try several)
$^1/_4$ c. chopped parsley
pinch herbs, thyme or rosemary
1 bay leaf

Simmer peas and water until soft (1–2 hours). Add other ingredients and boil gently for 10 minutes. Dilute to desired consistency with water as soup is blended in blender. Salt and season. Serve with **Croutons**. Serves 6.

Asparagus Soup

3–6 c. fresh asparagus: may use ends that
    are usually discarded
1 c. water
$^1/_4$ c. flour

3 c. **Soy or Nut Milk**
salt to taste
paprika for garnish

Cook asparagus in water until slightly tender. Transfer asparagus and water to blender and puree. If there are tough, fibrous strings, strain through a sieve. Mix remaining ingredients in blender and add to asparagus in saucepan. Simmer 5 minutes. Add a few cooked asparagus tips for color if desired. Adjust consistency with water or **Milk**. Salt to taste and garnish with paprika. Serve with **Melba Toast** or **Croutons**. Serves 4–5.

Corn Chowder

1 sliced onion
2 c. whole kernel corn
4 c. **Soy Milk**

4 potatoes, cooked in jackets,
    chopped

Whirl corn and **Soy Milk** in blender. Combine all ingredients and salt to taste, about $1^1/_4$ teaspoon. A sprinkle of chopped parsley on top is good. Serves 6.

Minestrone

$4^1/_2$ c. cooked beans
$^1/_2$ c. onion, chopped
10 c. water
1 c. uncooked **Spaghetti** broken in 1"
    pieces
2 t. salt

10 c. any vegetable or combination
    from the following list: **String
    Beans**, cabbage, tomatoes,
    eggplant, zucchini, celery,
    carrots, parsley

Combine ingredients and boil gently 30 to 45 minutes. Serves 12 to 15.

Bold Print indicates items listed in the INDEX

Chestnut Chutney

1 c. chopped chestnuts
1/2 c. raisins
1 t. vanilla, optional

salt if necessary
1 c. **Holiday Gravy or Basic Cream Sauce**

Mix together, heat, and serve as chutney over **Brown Rice** or **Millet** as a main dish at a fruit meal. Serves 4.

Seed Powder

Save all seeds removed from melons, squash, or similar vegetables. Particles of the vegetable which cling to seeds should not be removed as they add a nice flavor. Dry seeds in oven at about 275° until lightly browned. Grind to a powder in a seed mill. Use in many ways, such as scattered over desserts, sprinkled over the whipped topping as a garnish, or spooned over cereal to add body. Use in a salt shaker for vegetables, soups, or salads. **Popcorn** rejects may be ground for similar use.

Sunflower Seed Roast

4 c. water
1 c. sunflower seed
1 1/2 t. salt
1 t. celery salt

1 T. food yeast
1 c. onions, chopped
3 c. rolled oats

Blend the first five ingredients. Pour into bowl and add onions and oats. Let stand for 30 minutes or more. Pour into a floured baking dish, cover with foil, and bake for 45 minutes at 350°. Uncover, brown 20 minutes or more. Let cool to set before cutting. Final browning may be done next day if roast is prepared ahead of time and reheated. Serves 6.

Sunflower Loaf

1 c. bread crumbs
1/2 c. grated raw potato **or** chopped tomato
2 1/2 c. water

1/4 c. grated onion
1/2 c. ground sunflower seed
1 c. rolled oats
1 t. salt

Mix well. Bake for 1 hour at 350°. Serve with gravy. Serves 3–4.

Bold Print indicates items listed in the INDEX

V. ENTREES AND NUT MAIN DISHES

Roasted Nuts

The secret of properly roasted nuts is low oven temperature. Spread nuts in flat pans. Place in oven at 210° to 275°. Leave in overnight at 210°. Leave in 2–3 hours at 275°. Watch carefully during the last hour and stir if necessary. Use **Roasted Nuts** as **Main Dish**, about 1/4 cup, or as a side dish, 1–3 teaspoons.

Bologna

1/2 c. ground nuts	1/2 c. whole grain flour
3 c. fine **Cracker** crumbs	2 t. celery salt
2 c. water	2 t. salt
1 c. **Nut Milk**	1/4 t. sage

Whirl all the ingredients together in blender. Pour into large, floured, soup cans and steam or bake at 300° for 2 hours. Chill and slice thinly. Use in sandwiches with **Wheatonnaise** and **Alfalfa Sprouts**.

Homemade Hotdogs

1 c. grits, stoneground best	1 t. salt
2 c. water	1/4 c. finely chopped nuts
1 c. beet juice	1/4 t. mixed herbs
1 c. onions	

Whirl water, beet juice, onions, and salt in blender. Pour into nuts and grits. Boil together for 1 hour. Cool until grits begin to get slightly stiff. It is important not to overcool. Add herbs consisting of a mixture of about equal parts of sage and paprika. Spoon onto platters in hotdog shaped mounds measuring about 4″ × 3/4″. Allow to set by cooling. Roll in wheat germ. Bake at 425° for 30 to 60 minutes. Toast 1 minute under broiler if browning is desired. Serve with **Whole Wheat Buns**, **Mustard**, and **Catsup**. Makes 1–2 dozen hotdogs.

Dry Roasted Nuts

1 c. peanuts, or other nuts	1 1/2 T. starch
1 T. Karo or honey, optional	1/2 t. salt
1–2 T. water	

Mix all ingredients except peanuts. Pour over the peanuts and stir well to coat all the nuts. Bake slowly at 275° for 2–3 hours. Instead of honey, may use 1/2 teaspoon garlic powder or onion powder.

Bold Print indicates items listed in the INDEX

VI. RICE DISHES

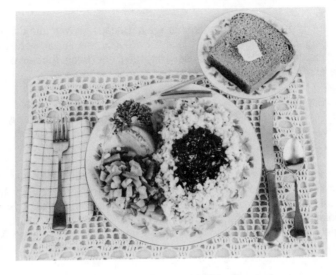

VI. RICE DISHES

INTRODUCTION

The world produces more rice than any other grain. Because it was found that rice keeps better for shipping and storage when polished, white rice has largely replaced brown or natural rice. This is a great pity because white rice has been robbed of much of its nutrient value and flavor.

Rice is good in puddings and desserts. It may be used to extend various foods. Add a few raisins to **Creamy Rice** and top it with grated coconut or whipped soy topping and you have a dessert to delight children. Rice served simply with a **Butter** or cream will go with any kind of meal. It provides an important standby for the cook.

Rice is highly nutritious and easily digested, being almost completely assimilated. It is the least allergenic of all foods. When it is milled so that only the husks are removed, the product is whole, brown, or natural rice. **Brown Rice** contains about 8% protein of very good biologic value, little fat, and 79% carbohydrate (chiefly starch). It has a good supply of minerals, including calcium, phosphorus, iron, and copper traces. The vitamins include B_1, B_2, niacin, and E. There are many essential micronutrients.

If the milling of rice is carried beyond removal of husks, the next step involves grinding away several outer layers of the grain to produce white rice. The by-products of this process are rice bran and rice polishings. They are used mostly in livestock feed. Rice bran and polishings contain 12% protein of a high biologic value.

Bold Print indicates items listed in the INDEX

VI. RICE DISHES

Risotto Milanese

$^1/_2$ c. chopped onion
2 crushed buds garlic
$1^1/_2$ c. brown rice
6 c. water **or** vegetable broth

1 t. basil
$1^1/_2$ t. salt
$^1/_2$ t. saffron steeped in 3 T. hot water, **or** 1 t. paprika

Dextrinize the rice in a dry skillet on low heat for about 8 minutes, stirring continuously. Add the broth very carefully with the basil, onion, garlic, and salt. Add the drained saffron after it has steeped in the hot water 15 minutes, or if saffron is not available use paprika. Cook the rice slowly for about 1–2 hours. Add more broth if necessary. Serve with **Sour Cream** or **Tomato Catsup**.

Dry Rice

1 c. brown rice
3 c. water

$1^1/_2$ t. salt

Heat the water, add the washed rice and the salt. Cook very slowly, covered, for $1^1/_4$ hours without stirring. Turn out into a serving bowl by rimming with a spatula and dumping to avoid crushing the grains. This makes **Fluffy Rice**. If desired, may cook in the top of a double boiler over boiling water for 3 hours. If it is to be served as a main dinner dish it may be stirred often to develop the creamy consistency of mashed potatoes. If served as breakfast rice, sweeten with some raisins and serve with **Sour Cream**. It may be piled into a casserole dish and kept hot in the oven, first sprinkling with a little chopped nuts. Serves 4.

Rice Balls

Press **Creamy Rice** into balls with hands after dipping into salted water (1 teaspoon per pint). Place on floured baking sheet and bake for 10 minutes at 450°. A small piece of fruit or vegetables or a nut may be enclosed in the center of each ball. May roll in wheat germ before baking.

Bold Print indicates items listed in the INDEX

VI. RICE DISHES

Rice with Pistachios, Pine Nuts, or Peanuts

2½ c. brown rice
1 onion
1 bud garlic
1½ t. paprika

½ c. pistachios
1¼ t. salt
5 c. water

Cook the rice, salt, and water, very slowly for 1½ hours. Chop the onion and garlic fine. Mix with nuts and paprika and stir into the rice. Cook 20 minutes. This is a good main dish for either breakfast or dinner. Serves 6.

Jamaica Rice and "Peas"

1¼ c. red kidney beans
4 c. water
1 T. salt
3 c. onions, chopped
1 T. lemon juice

1 T. mixed herbs
1 T. Karo
2⅓ c. raw brown rice
6½ c. water
2 buds garlic, minced

Wash beans and soak overnight. Cook 1 hour in soaking water, until beans crush easily between the fingers. Add the remaining ingredients and cook 2–3 hours more. If cooked well this is one of the finest rice dishes any country has produced. The Jamaicans call red kidney beans "peas." Turn into a large casserole, and bake slowly for 1 hour, adding a little more broth if necessary. The rice should be moist but fluffy. Serve with **Crackers** and a green salad for a complete meal. Serves 8–10.

Spanish Rice

1 c. **Cooked Garbanzos**
3 c. cooked **Dry Rice**
½ c. onion
½ c. green pepper

¾ c. **Tomato Paste or** cooked
  tomatoes
2 c. water
2 T. soy flour
½ t. onion salt

Chop onion and pepper. Mix and add last 4 items. Simmer gently until thickened, about 3–5 minutes. Add **Rice** and **Garbanzos**. Bake in floured casserole 25 minutes at 350°. Serves 4. Variation: Substitute green peas for the **Garbanzos**.

Rice Pie

Add 10 to 20% sautéed or leftover vegetables to cooked rice. Make creamy with vegetable broth, water or **Soy Milk**. Pile in a baking dish and ice with **Mashed Potatoes**. Bake in very hot oven until peaks are a golden brown.

Bold Print indicates items listed in the INDEX

"Saffron" Rice

1 c. brown rice, dextrinized if desired
1 c. chopped baked sweet potato
$1/2$ c. onions

$1/4$ t. ground coriander
3 c. water
1 t. salt

Place all ingredients except rice in blender until smooth. Put rice in a kettle and pour in the blended ingredients. Cover and cook without stirring for 1–2 hours. Serves 4.

Sesame Rice

3 c. **Creamy Rice**

$1/3$ c. ground, roasted, unhulled, sesame seed

Stir sesame seed into rice, stirring vigorously to cream. Use as a breakfast cereal with a **Fruit Sauce**, or as a main dish for dinner with boiled cabbage wedges and sliced tomatoes. Serves 3.

Rice Meal

4 c. **Creamy Rice**
2 c. **Cooked Garbanzos**

1 c. sautéed onions
salt as needed

Mix ingredients and place in a baking dish. Heat thoroughly at 350° for about 20 to 30 minutes before serving. Serves 4. With a green salad makes a complete meal.

Flaky Rice

1 c. rice
$2^1/2$ c. water

$1/2$ t. salt

Toast rice in a dry pan on burner while stirring constantly or in oven at 350° for 15 to 20 minutes until turning golden and rice begins to pop. Pour immediately into preheated water. Use care as water will boil vigorously as the toasted rice is poured in. Reduced heat to a bare simmer for 1–2 hours. Do not stir during any of the cooking period even though some sticks to the bottom. When finished cooking and all kernels are soft and well cooked, turn out carefully onto a platter to prevent its becoming creamy. It is better to cook **Flaky Rice** in a large flat pan such as an electric fry pan rather than a small diameter, deep kettle, as the deeper layers tend to get more creamy as the depth of the rice increases. To remove the crust which may sometimes stick to the bottom, simply add a small amount of water and cover pot for a few minutes. Then lift the crust out with a spatula. Cut the crust in wedges and serve as wafers.

Rice Powder or Flour

Dextrinize brown rice by roasting in a dry skillet stirring constantly until golden and it begins to pop, or place in 350° oven for 15 to 20 minutes. Blend at high speed until it becomes a powder, or grind fine in a mill. Use for thickening stews and gravies, as a binder in casseroles, and for **Rice Cream**.

VI. RICE DISHES

MISCELLANEOUS RICE ITEMS

Creamy Rice

1 c. rice
3 c. water

$^1/_2$ t. salt

Place ingredients in a pressure cooker at 5 pounds for 30 minutes or a covered kettle for 2–3 hours. Stir vigorously before removing to make creamy. Use in any recipe needing a rich body such as stews, pudding, or casseroles. Use also as a breakfast cereal with a fruit topping. Serves about 4.

Cream of Rice
"Rice Cream"

1 c. **Rice Powder**
3–4 c. water

$^1/_2$ t. salt

Sauté **Rice Powder** sprinkled over the bottom of a kettle until the powder has a nut-like fragrance. Cool the powder by setting the pan in cold water. Add the water gradually, stirring constantly to prevent lumping. Add salt. Cook in covered kettle for about 20 minutes. Stir vigorously to mix before serving. Wheat or rye flour may be treated in the same way. Serve with fruit as a breakfast dish, or stir in cubed avocado, cucumber, or tomatoes as a dinner dish. May be thinned with broth and poured over green beans or dried beans as a gravy. Yield: 4 cups.

Paella-Limas
(pie-el-ya)

2 c. brown rice
4$^1/_2$ c. boiling water
1 c. green limas

1 large carrot, sliced thin
1 t. salt
1 large onion, minced

Dextrinize rice in a heavy skillet until slightly brown and popping. Sauté onions and carrots together in a little water for 3 minutes. Pour all ingredients into boiling water and boil for 30 minutes. Pour the **Paella** into a casserole, cover and bake at 350° for 1 hour. Leave uncovered last 5 minutes. Serve with a green salad for a complete meal. Serves 6–8.

Bold Print indicates items listed in the INDEX

Rice and Soybean Loaf

1$^1/_2$ c. cooked soybeans	3 T. water, **or** broth
1 c. **Flaky Rice**	salt to taste
$^1/_4$ c. flour	herbs and onion, optional

Place the boiled, drained soybeans in a blender with 3 tablespoons of broth, having the puree as dry as possible. Sauté the flour in a dry pan until a nut-like aroma forms. Add to soy puree and mix with the cooked rice. Salt to taste, pack in floured brick-shaped loaf pan, and bake at 350° until nicely browned, about 50 minutes. May be made into patties $^3/_4$″ thick and baked 20–30 minutes at 350° until crusty brown. Serves 4.

Lentil and Rice Loaf

2 c. **Dry Rice**	3 T. water
1 c. **Lentil Puree**	a sprinkle of sage
1 T. chopped onion	salt to taste
$^1/_3$ c. chopped walnuts	2 T. whole grain flour, browned

Mix all the ingredients. Pack lightly in a floured bread tin, and bake at 350° about 45 minutes until slightly browned on top. Serves 4.

Stuffed Cabbage

8–10 large green cabbage leaves	$^1/_2$ c. minced onion
3 c. cooked rice	1 t. salt
$^1/_2$ c. ground cashews	$^2/_3$ c. stewed tomatoes
$^1/_2$ c. chopped parsley	

Parboil the whole cabbage leaves until soft. Mix all other items. Place about $^1/_2$ cup of the rice mixture on each cabbage leaf. Roll up and secure each leaf with a skewer or toothpick and bake in covered casserole 45 minutes at 375°. Serves 3–4. Serve with **Sour Cream**.

Bold Print indicates items listed in the INDEX

VI. RICE DISHES

Persian Baked Rice

1 c. brown rice with 2½ c. water   1 onion
⅛ t. ground coriander   1 t. salt

Wash the rice and put it in a casserole which has a tight lid. Put the onion in the center of the rice. Boil up the water with the coriander and salt and add it to the rice. Cover tightly and bake 2 hours at 325°. Remove onion. If rice is not perectly dry and fluffy, lift gently with a fork and let it stay 15 minutes in the oven with the lid removed. This is a fine way to cook rice, and especially nice to serve with oriental dishes and with **Apricot Sauce**. Rice baked this way can be mixed with custards for breakfast or desserts if onion is omitted. Serves 3 or 4.

Tomato and Okra Pilau

1½ c. brown rice	1–2 c. okra, cut in 1″ lengths
1 c. water	3–5 c. tomatoes **or** 5–10 tomatoes
2 large onions, sliced thin	salt
1 green pepper, diced	1 t. Karo

Boil the washed brown rice in 1 cup of water for 12 minutes. Sauté the okra, onion, and pepper in water until tender. If fresh tomatoes are used, skin and slice them. Combine all the ingredients, cover and cook slowly about 1 hour or until the rice is tender and has absorbed the juice from the tomatoes. Turn into a hot dish and sprinkle the top with chopped green onions if desired. Serves 6.

Rice Pudding

4 c. cooked **Rice**	½ t. salt
⅓ c. whole grain flour	½ c. raisins
1 c. **Soy Milk**, **Nut Milk**, **or Basic**	1 t. ground coriander
Cream Sauce	2–4 T. Karo **or** honey

Mix ingredients. Use 2 tablespoons honey if serving as breakfast dish, 4 if serving as dessert. Place in a casserole. Sprinkle the top with ground nuts if desired. Bake at 350° for 60 minutes. Serves 4–6.

Bold Print indicates items listed in the INDEX

VII. GRAVIES & SAUCES

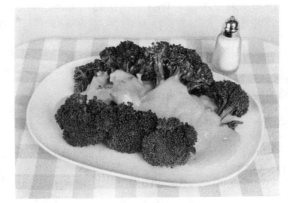

VII. GRAVIES AND SAUCES

INTRODUCTION

Sauces are more than just gravy. They may be sweet, to serve with desserts and break-fast foods such as cereals, waffles, and toasts. (See the section on "**Cereal**, **Waffle**, and **Dessert Toppings**, **Spreads**.") Sauce may also be subtly flavored and smooth, to serve with roasts, patties, or soufflés. The purpose of fine sauce is to enhance the flavors of the dish it accompanies, not cover up or alter.

If the basic sauces are learned, it is easy to become proficient in making many good sauces. To make masterpieces of simple dishes requires only a light touch with the onion, the flour, the broth or cream; then the final fillip which makes the difference between good and excellent—the seasoning, consisting of herbs, food yeast, flavorings, etc.

The first basic sauce is the **Cream Sauce**. One must learn to make a roux first, blending and lightly browning the flour. Slowly add the liquid, and stir continuously. Simmer 3 or 4 minutes over a very low flame to cook the flour. If sauces are made without hurry they will be creamy and smooth. Never have sauces too thick when they are served; and never have so much that the food is swimming in it.

Spices and herbs include a variety of vegetable products which are aromatic and have pungent flavors. They are used to enhance the natural flavors of foods. Many herbs add certain of the trace elements to the daily dietary. Many of these trace elements are dif-ficult to obtain from any other source. The use of herbs is rewarding from more than one aspect.

Herbs are from the leafy parts of the temperate zone plants. Certain non-toxic seeds may also be used to flavor foods. Care to avoid any irritating herb will be richly repaid in good health of the stomach. Herbs gradually lose flavor and color during storage. They should not be purchased in large quantity. Store them in a cool, dry place in airtight containers to retard loss of flavor. If you are unfamiliar with an herb, test its effect on different foods by using a small quantity in a recipe at first, about $1/4$ teaspoon per pint or pound of food. The flavor needs to blend in certain foods, and to be kept distinct in certain others. If the first effect is desired, add the flavor at the beginning of the preparation. If the flavor is to be kept separate from the food it is used with, add just before serving or pass around in a shaker.

Spices are defined as parts of plants, such as the seeds, buds, fruit, flowers, bark or roots of plants, usually of tropical origin. They are sold whole or ground. Several spices are irritating to the stomach and to the nerves. These irritating spices should be avoided.

Safe Herbs

Basil	Fennel Seed	Onion	Saffron
Bay Leaf	Garlic	Paprika	Sage
Coriander	Marjoram	Parsley	Sesame Seed
Dill Seed	Mint	Rosemary	Tarragon
			Thyme

Bold Print indicates items listed in the INDEX

Irritating Substances

NAME	CHEMICAL	EFFECT
Black pepper	Eugenol	GI* and GU* irritation, ↑ BP*
Chili peppers		↑ Cancer, ↑ BP*
Cayenne		Stomach irritation
Horseradish		GU* irritation
Cloves		↑ Cravings, irritates nerves
Cinnamon		↑ Cravings, irritates nerves
Mustard seed	Allyl oil	GU* irritation, ↑ BP*
Ginger		GU* irritation, ↑ BP*
Nutmeg	Myristicin	Breaks mucus barriers in stomach and bowel, hallucinations, may depress or irritate central nervous system
Hungarian paprika		GI* irritation
Vinegar	Acetic acid	Breaks mucus barriers, irritates nerves
Baking soda, powder	Sodium salts	↑ BP*, ↑ stomach irritation
Salt	Sodium chloride	↑ BP*, ↑ cravings

*GI: Gastrointestinal
*GU: Genitourinary

*BP: Blood Pressure
Arrows indicate increase

Curry, Nonirritating

1 T. paprika
1 T. dill seed

1 T. ground coriander
1 T. garlic powder

Mix. Store tightly closed. Use in any recipe calling for curry.

Chicken Style Seasoning

1 c. food yeast
2$^1/_2$ t. sweet pepper flakes, powdered
3 t. onion powder
3$^1/_2$ t. salt
2$^1/_2$ t. sage

2$^1/_2$ t. thyme
2$^1/_2$ t. garlic powder
1$^1/_4$ t. marjoram
1$^1/_4$ t. rosemary

Mix. May omit or add ingredients. Store tightly closed.

Bold Print indicates items listed in the INDEX

VII. GRAVIES AND SAUCES

Seasoned Gravy

2 c. water
$1/4$ c. brown flour
$1/2$ t. salt

1 t. onion powder
$1/4$ t. any mixed herbs

Liquefy and cook until done (about 10 minutes). Serve with vegetarian roasts or burgers, and as stock for many stews, casseroles, and baked vegetables. Serves 6.

Holiday Gravy

3 c. water
$1/2$ c. flour, **dextrinized**

1 T. **food yeast**
1 t. salt

Place flour in dry pan in oven at 300° for about 10 to 15 minutes to lightly brown (dextrinize). Since barley is used infrequently elsewhere, it is well to use barley flour for gravies to increase the variety of grains used. Barley flour is mild flavored and light in color. Make flour in blender from pearl barley. Mix all ingredients in a blender and cook in a saucepan, stirring until thickened, then cover and simmer for about 10 minutes. Serves 8–10.

Cashew Gravy

2 c. water
$1/4$ c. cashews **or** other nuts
$1/4$ c. flour **or** 2 T. starch

$1/2$ t. salt
1 t. onion powder **or** medium onion

Place all ingredients in blender until fine. Cook over medium heat until flour is thickened, stirring constantly. Cover and allow to simmer 10 minutes. To alter flavor, use barley or rye flour browned lightly in oven. Serves 6.

Peanut Butter Gravy

$1^1/2$ c. water
$1/2$–$3/4$ c. peanut butter
$1/2$ c. white **or** whole wheat flour **or**
      $1/4$ c. corn starch
$1^1/2$ t. salt

1 t. onion powder
1 t. sweet basil or celery seed
1 T. Chicken Style Seasoning,
      optional

Blend smooth and pour into $2^1/2$ cup of boiling water in a saucepan, while stirring. Continue to stir until it comes to a boil again. Cook flour 20 minutes, and starch until thick.

Bold Print indicates items listed in the INDEX

VII. GRAVIES AND SAUCES

Coconut Gravy

2 c. water
$^1/_2$ c. unsweetened shredded coconut

2 T. starch
$^1/_2$ t. salt

Liquefy the ingredients for 1 minute in a blender. Cook for 3–5 minutes, stirring constantly. Use over cereals instead of milk. Very good as a topping for desserts. Dilute slightly and use over **Baked Sweet Potato** or winter squash such as butternut or acorn. May be used as a spread on bread instead of mayonnaise in sandwiches using fruit such as bananas or pineapple. Variation: Add 1–2 tablespoons lemon juice for a tart gravy. Serves 6.

Brown Gravy

$^1/_2$ c. whole grain flour
2 c. vegetable broth **or** water

salt to taste

Put the flour in a fry pan, heat while dry, stirring constantly to **Dextrinize** and develop a nut-like odor. When entirely browned, cool slightly by rubbing pan with a wet cloth. Add one third of the liquid, and stir until smooth and, free from lumps. Add the rest of the liquid, and let boil slowly for 10 minutes. For variation, sauté chopped onions in a little water, or add chopped olives just before serving. If smooth texture is desired, return to blender and blend until creamy. Serves 6.

Tomato Gravy

1 pt. tomatoes
1 small onion, chopped fine
$^1/_2$ clove garlic
2 stalks celery chopped fine

1 t. salt
$^1/_4$ c. whole grain flour
$^1/_4$ c. cold water

Simmer the first four items 5 minutes. Make a paste using the flour and water. Add to the tomatoes. Simmer slowly over very low heat for 10 to 20 minutes. One half bay leaf may be added if desired. If a smooth gravy is preferred whirl in blender just before serving. Serves 6.

Bean Gravy

Use any leftover beans, peas, split peas, lentils, or garbanzos. Place 1–2 cups in blender with enough water or **Soy Milk** (base or milk) to make the desired consistency. Season with onion or garlic, salt and herbs. Good on **Grits**, **Rice**, and **Melba Toast**.

Bold Print indicates items listed in the INDEX

VII. GRAVIES AND SAUCES

GRAVIES

Basic Gravy and Custard Recipe

4 c. water   1 t. salt
1 c. brown flour

Mix ingredients and cook gently until thick. Reduce flame and barely simmer for 20 minutes. May be thinned with vegetable broth, **Soy**, or **Nut Milk**, or fruit juice in the case of custards. May add nuts, **Nut Butters**, or seeds for a more rich gravy or custard. One recipe serves about 10 as gravy, or about 6 as cereal topping. Optional seasonings: Onion, garlic, herbs, seasoning salts (omit salt). May use flavorings such as banana, lemon, orange, vanilla, etc. with $1/4$ cup Karo for a custard topping for cereals.

Almond Gravy

$1^1/_2$ c. water   1 T. yeast flakes
$1/_2$ c. white flour or $1/_4$ c. corn starch $1^1/_2$ t. onion powder
$1/_4$ c. cashews, almonds, ground fine   2 t. **Chicken Style Seasoning**
                                      1 t. salt

Blend smooth and pour into $2^1/_2$ c. boiling water in a saucepan, stirring constantly until it boils again. Add $3/_4$ cup chopped or slivered almonds.

Rice Gravy

1 c. cooked rice or millet, hot   2 t. **Chicken Style Seasoning**
$1/_4$ c. almonds or cashews, **or** 2–3 T.   2 c. hot water or vegetable broth
      peanut butter   salt to taste

Blend smooth. Pour into a saucepan and heat, stirring constantly. Simmer gently a few minutes. Makes about 3 cups.

Bold Print indicates items listed in the INDEX

Basic Cream Sauce

	THIN	MEDIUM	THICK
Whole wheat flour	2 T.	3 T.	4 T.
Unbleached white flour	1 T.	2 T.	3 T.
Rye	2 T.	3 T.	4 T.
Starch	1 T.	2 T.	3 T.
Arrowroot flour	2 t.	1½ T.	2 T.
Rice flour	2 t.	1½ T.	2 T.
Barley flour	2 T.	3 T.	4 T.
Salt	¼ t.	¼ t.	½ t.
Water	1 c.	1 c.	1 c.
Soy Base	¼ c.	¼ c.	¼ c.

Liquefy in blender. Cook over low fire, stirring constantly until thick and thoroughly cooked. Use thin cream sauce for soups, medium for scalloped or creamed dishes, and thick for croquettes. May use as a broth to cook vegetables.

Bold Print indicates items listed in the INDEX

VII. GRAVIES AND SAUCES

Vegetable Dressing

1 fresh vegetable
1 T. lemon juice

$\frac{1}{2}$ t. salt
water as needed

Put a succulent vegetable such as a tomato in blender with the seasonings and whirl at high speed until smooth. If onions, pepper, cucumber, radishes, or other vegetables are used, water may be needed in the blender to develop the whirling. Serve over any vegetable salad.

Lemon and Onion Dressing

Put a few tablespoons of lemon juice in blender. Add fresh onion. Blend until smooth. Use as dressing.

Soyonnaise—Oil Free

2 c. hot water
$\frac{2}{3}$ c. Soyagen
$\frac{1}{2}$ c. hot rice

1 t. salt
$\frac{1}{2}$ t. dill weed, optional
1 t. **Chicken Style Seasoning**

Blend very smooth and stir in $\frac{1}{4}$ cup lemon juice. Chill and serve.

Cashew Mayonnaise

$\frac{1}{2}$ c. cashews
$1\frac{1}{2}$ c. water, boiling

1 t. salt
$\frac{1}{2}$ t. onion powder

Blend, cook, stirring constantly, then add 2–4 tablespoon lemon juice.

Bold Print indicates items listed in the INDEX

VII. GRAVIES AND SAUCES

Fine Herbs Sauce

2 T. chopped onion
1 T. chopped parsley
1 bay leaf
$1/_4$ c. water
1 T. flour

2 c. canned tomatoes
$1/_2$ c. vegetable broth **or** water
1 T. lemon juice
$1/_2$ t. salt

Braise the first four ingredients for a few minutes. Add the flour and stir. Whirl the remaining items in blender until smooth. Add to the onion mixture and let simmer for 10 minutes. Remove the bay leaf as soon as the sauce is flavored to taste.

Tomato Sauce

Drain canned tomatoes or fresh, peeled tomatoes and whirl in blender to make smooth. Place in oven in a large flat pan to concentrate while baking other foods. When evaporation has caused thickening to the consistency of sauce, pour up into a storage container. Keeps 2–3 weeks in the refrigerator. Do not allow storage container to warm up but remove a small quantity as needed. May be frozen up to one year.

Tomato Paste

Proceed as for **Tomato Sauce**, but continue the evaporation process until the consistency of paste is achieved.

Golden Sauce
(see **Cheese** Recipes, page 52)

Tomato French Dressing

4–6 c. cooked tomatoes
1 t. salt
1 t. onion powder
$1/_2$ t. sweet basil
$1/_2$ t. dill

$1/_4$ t. celery seed
$1/_4$ t. garlic powder
1 T. lemon
1 T. turbinado sugar

Blend. Serve over salads, roasts, rice or noodles, or as soup.

Bold Print indicates items listed in the INDEX

VII. GRAVIES AND SAUCES

SAUCES

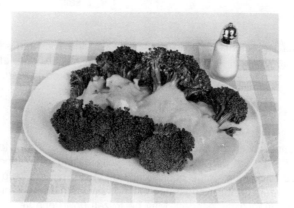

Golden Sauce served over **Broccoli**

VIII. SALAD DRESSINGS, SANDWICH, & BURGER SPREADS

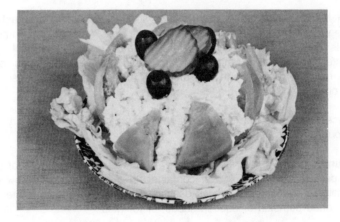

PROPER USE OF THE BLENDER

1. Put liquid portions of recipies into blender container before dry ingredients to prevent sticking to bottom.

2. Cut all fruits and vegetables in 1″ pieces before blending for greatest ease in processing.

3. Place cover firmly on container before starting or stopping to prevent jumping out. May remove cover in mid-cycle.

4. If blender blades throw processing food up so that the whirlpool effect stops and blades begin to whiz ineffectually, remove cover with motor running, and push the ingredients from sides to center with a rubber spatula until the whirlpool again forms. Then move the spatula up and down rapidly, tight against the sides to avoid the blades. It may be necessary to turn motor off for a moment to release the bubble of air which is caught in the blades.

5. Don't process mixtures too long or overtax the motor with extra heavy loads such as stiff doughs.

6. Make **Crumbs** from whole grain **Breads** or **Crackers** by tearing fresh or dried bread into 5–6 pieces, placing in blender container for a few seconds at low or medium speed until the crumb is as fine as desired. The same process is fine for leftover **Popcorn**, dried pumpkin or squash seeds, or for nuts.

7. Grains or beans may be ground into flour or grits by the method described in 6.

8. Dried or fresh citrus peel may be grated at high speeds. To dry peel, place in oven at 200° until no trace of moisture is left and peel is crisp but not toasted. Store in freezer up to one year.

9. Batter, **Nut Butters**, **Nut Milk**, and drinks may be made easily in the blender. See recipes given.

10. To liquefy raw vegetables such as carrots, cube and barely cover with water. Process until smooth.

Bold Print indicates items listed in the INDEX

IRRITATING FOODS

Many spreads depend on vinegar to give a certain desirable sourness. Yet vinegar is an irritant both to the delicate linings of the intestinal tract and to the nerves. In this fast age we live in, the less irritating and exciting our food the better will be the health of our population. Condiments are injurious in their very chemistry. The blood is made impure and of an irritating chemical quality by the pickles, spices, peppery foods, mustard, and mayonnaise type spreads and dressings. The ingredients of many condiments have been associated with the production of cancer of the digestive organs. It is possible to prepare tasty, simple spreads, dressings, and sauces as companions for bread, vegetables, pastas and other foods without using a single injurious chemical. Lemon juice can easily take the place of vinegar. Various harmless herbs can supply the place of irritating spices. With the use of labor-saving devices such as blenders and seed mills, there are many blends of lemon juice with cooked cereal bases that can give your dishes a gourmet quality, either sweet or savory.

Many individuals, both children and adults, are being made nervous by the foods they eat and the beverages they drink. Most kitchens have bottles and jars of fiery foods, sauces, and pickles that are placed on the table with each meal. The family members and guests partake freely of these irritating foods which cause a delicate constitution and a nervousness that the person does not understand. It is all the more perplexing if some members of the family do not seem to suffer digestive complaints from eating the highly spiced or seasoned foods. The same foods eaten by the various family members may cause a short temper in one, a peptic ulcer in another, depression in yet another, and fatigue and sleeplessness in another. The family is afflicted, yet the cause is unsuspected. Habits of eating, drinking, and dressing can greatly affect the health and productivity of the family.

Excitement of the taste buds by stimulating foods is sought because, for the time, the results are agreeable. But the overuse of the electrical pathways in the nervous system brings a reaction in all cases. The use of stimulating food and drink always tends to excess. They are active agents in bringing on degenerative diseases. The cook should not feel at liberty to prepare dishes that are exciting or that tempt to excess.

Bold Print indicates items listed in the INDEX

Soy Spread

$^1/_3$ c. soy flour
$^1/_3$ c. white flour
1$^3/_4$ c. water
$^1/_2$ t. salt

2 T. lemon juice
$^1/_4$ t. garlic powder
1 t. honey

Dextrinize the flours together for 15 minutes at 300°. Mix with the water and cook gently, stirring constantly for the first 3 minutes. Reduce heat and simmer for 10 minutes. Add remaining ingredients, stirring well. Store in refrigerator up to two weeks. Whip with a fork to make smooth when ready to serve. May need to add some water if too thick. Use as a sandwich spread or as a salad dressing, in the same way mayonnaise is used.

Wheatonnaise
Using Wheat Flour

1 c. water
$^1/_2$ c. ground cashews, optional

$^1/_4$ c. wheat flour

Whirl in blender. Boil 5 minutes, stirring constantly. Cool and return to blender.

$^1/_2$ c. raw carrots **or** apples
$^1/_2$ t. salt
1 T. honey
1 clove garlic **or** onion (optional, omit when **Wheatonnaise** is to be used as **Sour Cream** with fruit dishes, or as **Whipped Topping**)

$^1/_2$ c. water
1 T. lemon juice

Add all ingredients to blender. Whirl until smooth.

Pimiento Cream

Mix the following items with a fork: 2 tablespoons pimiento puree (made by whirling pimientos in blender) and $^1/_2$ cup **Wheatonnaise**. Do not use blender to mix as it will lose body. Spoon onto **Soups** as a garnish, or serve over **Greens**, **Grits**, beans, or **Burgers**.

Bold Print indicates items listed in the INDEX

French Dressing

1/4 c. lemon juice	Optional seasonings:
1 t. salt	fennel powder
2 t. paprika	tarragon
1 c. canned tomatoes, blended	basil
	garlic, crushed
	Karo **or** honey
	dill

Mix all ingredients in a blender. Season the dressing for variety. If fresh herbs are not available, very good aromatic dried ones are generally obtainable. A supply of dressing may be kept in the refrigerator in a jar.

CONCENTRATED FOODS

It has been found that laboratory animals will not partake of most of the rich and complicated mixtures that humans eat freely. The less we place condiments, fried foods, and desserts on our tables the better it will be for all, both active and sedentary of lifestyle. Rich foods are health destroying. Foods can be made rich in a number of different ways. The addition of any concentrated food or refined food element makes food rich. Oils, nuts, wheat germ, sugar or honey, food yeast, coconut, various seeds, olives, and many other heavy or concentrated foods can make rich dishes.

Not only rich foods but also complicated foods are injurious to the health of human beings. The cook must exert care at all times against the tendency to make dishes more and more complex. In making salads, often two or more leafy items will be added, then bell pepper and tomatoes, a generous grating of carrots or other tubers, then olives, legumes, and nuts may be thrown in. Many take pride in making salads more and more complex, and feel that they are carrying out the principles of good nutrition. The fact is that the greater the combination of foods the more likely the dish is to set up a war inside of one. Both in the digestive tract and in the blood there is an unhealthy competition for carrier systems, adsorption sites, and biochemical pathways. We can indeed say that, "All mixed and complicated foods are injurious to the health of human beings." E. G. White, COUNSELS ON DIET AND FOODS, page 113.

In a manner similar to that of making salads, casseroles and roasts are often made of bits of many foods that have been left from another meal. If possible the "Russian style" of serving, in which all the food is served out, should be used for foods that could present troublesome leftovers. With this style of serving there are no leftovers. It may be that only certain dishes will be served out and others such as bread, rice, whole fruits, or vegetables which present no problem if there are leftovers, can be served family style. The Russian style of serving also helps to prevent overeating.

Bold Print indicates items listed in the INDEX

LOW CALORIE DRESSINGS

Zero Dressing

1 part tomato juice
1 part lemon juice
salt

Seasonings (dill, onion, chives,
    garlic, celery, cucumber,
    paprika, parsley, food yeast)

Blend lightly. Refrigerate. Use on salads, roasts, breads. Shake well before using.

French Dressing
Low Calorie

1 c. water or tomato juice
$1/4$–$1/2$ c. lemon juice
1 t. honey

$1/2$–2 t. paprika
$1/2$ t. salt, if needed
1 t. onion **or** garlic salt
$1/2$ t. dill

Shake together in a jar. Refrigerate.

Mustard Lo-Cal

1 clove garlic
$1/2$ c. lemon juice
$1/2$ c. water
$1^1/4$ c. raw or cooked carrots

$1/2$ t. paprika
$1/2$ t. salt
$1/4$ c. unbleached white flour

Put last four ingredients in blender to mix. Cook about 10 minutes. Return to blender and add garlic and lemon juice. Whirl until smooth.

Catsup Lo-Cal

1 c. **Tomato Paste**
2 t. honey
1 t. salt

2 T. lemon juice
blended garlic **or** onion, as desired

Whiz until smooth.

Bold Print indicates items listed in the INDEX

IX. VEGETABLES

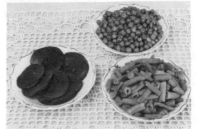

IX. VEGETABLES

ESSENTIAL FOUR FOOD GROUPS

As one of the essential four food groups, vegetables furnish a major portion of vitamins, proteins, and minerals. Most vegetables have oils and carbohydrates in varying quantities. The other three essential food groups are fruits, nuts, and grains. These four together furnish all the nutrients we need for development of growth, maintenance of health, and recovery from illness.

A WIDE VARIETY THE FIRST RULE OF NUTRITION

One should become accustomed to using as wide a variety as is possible. Use as many things in season as can be obtained. The closer the garden is to the table, both in time and distance, the more benefit we can derive from our food. Surplus food, however, should be carefully stored by canning, freezing, drying, or packing. Handle vegetables promptly after picking to avoid the loss of nutrients that come from long delays in processing, standing in sunshine, wilting, or softening. Paring, shredding, and slicing should be done immediately before use or processing to avoid nutrient losses. Vitamin C is especially vulnerable to loss.

COOLING PRINCIPLES

Steaming is a good way to cook vegetables without excessive loss of nutrients. Get about 20 holes of ¼" diameter bored in the upper section of a double boiler. Place vegetables in the upper section and boil water in the lower part. Do not crowd vegetables in the boiler, and salt just before serving.

Whenever possible, vegetables should be cooked and served the same day they are gathered. If necessary to store vegetables for a period, do not put them in water, as that will dissolve minerals and vitamins, and promote deterioration and spoilage. Store in a cold place. Stored vegetables should be immersed in cool water for 30 to 60 minutes before cooking to make them more tender.

Bicarbonate of soda should never be used as a color preserver for greens nor as a conditioner in cooking legumes and grains, as it destroys part of the nutritive value of the food. It leaves a harmful residue in the food.

In this chapter an effort is made to teach the best way to cook vegetables so they may show to their best advantage as to appearance, flavor and food value. Steamed or creamed vegetables can be beautiful to look at. What is more inviting than a casserole topped with molten gold of bubbling **Chee Sauce**! As most dinners are not complete without a vegetable, the cooking should be with care and understanding.

Fresh succulent vegetables should be cooked as little as possible. Over cooking toughens the texture of some vegetable foods, destroys the coloring, and damages the minerals that contribute to their flavor and nutritive value. Vegetables should be allowed to boil slowly. Rapid boiling hardens some foods. Steaming of vegetables hastens the cooking, shortens the time of meal preparation, and preserves the nutrients best. Use only sufficient water to produce the steam needed.

IX. VEGETABLES

Pressure cooking where possible is a saver of both time and nutrients. Use the following chart for cooking time of common vegetables.

GUIDE FOR BOILING VEGETABLES

This table is given merely as a rough guide. Any vegetable should be cooked only as long as necessary to develop flavor and desired consistency. The age, freshness, and size will determine cooking time.

VEGETABLE	COOKING TIME
Asparagus:	
tips	5–10 min.
stalks	20–25 min.
Beans, string	15–30 min.
Beets, young	20–60 min.
Beets, old	3–4 hours
Broccoli	15–25 min.
Brussels sprouts	9–10 min.
Cabbage	5–10 min.
Carrots, young	15–20 min.
Carrots, old	30–40 min.
Cauliflower	8–10 min.
Celery	15–20 min.
Collards	20–60 min.
Onions	25–35 min.
Parsnips	30–40 min.
Peas	10–15 min.
Potatoes:	
Irish	20–30 min.
sweet	20–25 min.
Rutabagas	25–30 min.
Squash:	
summer	5–20 min.
winter	30–45 min.
Spinach:	
with stems	6–10 min.
without stems	4–5 min.
Tomatoes	5–10 min.
Turnips	20–60 min.

The reason why greens, especially those fully grown, require more cooking than succulent vegetables, is that in growing for some time exposed to the sun, they develop a bitter flavor, and this is largely converted by the period of cooking. When spinach is very tender, it may be cooked with no additional water beyond that remaining on the leaves after washing. During the cooking, spinach should be turned over occasionally with a fork or a spoon, the saucepan being covered, to enclose the steam. It will require but a few minutes cooking. Serve spinach without chopping, but chop other greens well before serving.

Bold Print indicates items listed in the INDEX

IX. VEGETABLES

AVOID SPOILAGE OR FERMENTATION

There should be no food served on our tables that has the slightest taint of spoilage about it. Nor should any foods that have a rotting or fermenting stage in their processing be used. Sauerkraut is one of these foods. It is allowed to ferment for 3–4 weeks in a warm place, not below 70°. During this period foam and mildew must be removed from the top periodically and the top portion skimmed off and the cover washed free of the fermentation products. Unlike the rising process of bread which involves only the yeast, sugar, and water, the gluten serving only to trap the gas bubbles, the cabbage itself is involved in the fermentation process and is subjected to chemical change during the several weeks of processing. Hard cheese is also given a putrefying or "ripening" process of 1–5 weeks or more. Toxic amines and other chemicals accumulate causing this kind of cheese to be unfit for human consumption.

THE SUPERIOR LEAF PROTEIN

The leaf protein is nutritionally superior to most nut and seed proteins, as good as animal proteins, and can be presented at the table in many palatable forms. Leaf protein is one of the foodstuffs that can be used, especially in the wet tropics to ameliorate the protein shortage that now exists.

VEGETABLE COOKERY HINTS

IDEAL REQUIREMENTS FOR A COOKING PAN:

1. Have straight sides.
2. Have flat bottom.
3. Tight fitting lid.
4. Hard surfaces easily cleaned.
5. Hold and distribute heat evenly.

BEST METHODS FOR COOKING VEGETABLES:

1. Cook without water, if possible.
2. Cook as short a time as possible and just before serving.
3. Avoid bruising, soaking, or wilting vegetables.
4. Keep vegetables cold until ready to cook.
5. Avoid use of soda for preserving color and crispness.
6. Do not remove cover while cooking.
7. Avoid the use of utensils that are chipped, worn, or have copper alloys.
8. Use plastic scouring pad or stiff brush for vegetables, not a metal mesh pad.
9. When done, vegetables should have a crisp, tender texture. Overcooked they are mushy, strong flavored, and lose attractive natural color.

Bold Print indicates items listed in the INDEX

10. Cook vegetables whole or in large pieces when possible. Cook with skins on to save nutrients.
11. Start vegetables in boiling water to conserve the greatest possible amount of nutrients. To preserve the bright green color, cook vegetables uncovered for 1 minute AFTER boiling point has been reached, cover, reduce heat promptly to lowest cooking level, and cook until done.
12. Stir as little as possible, and do not boil vigorously.
13. A small amount of lemon juice added to the cooking water will help restore the color of red cabbage and beets.
14. Serve as soon as the vegetable is cooked. Keeping vegetables warm after they are cooked causes loss of food value, particularly vitamins. If they must wait, allow to cool, then reheat.

SEASONING VEGETABLES

There are many different ways to make vegetables taste well-seasoned without using salt or oil, and still avoiding harmful substances such as vinegar and black pepper or other spices. The good health principle of restricting salt intake to $1/2$ teaspoon per day makes those accustomed to more salt feel that the food is flat. For these persons the use of lemon juice perks up the food. Tomato can be used in a similar way, raw and chopped, canned, as **Sauce**, or as the puree. Onion and green pepper, celery, parsley, or garlic will add interesting touches. The addition of chopped nuts or **Ground Seeds** adds a delightful flavor to many foods. Use the leftover **Popcorn** kernels ground to a powder and added to potatoes, cereals, sweet potatoes, salads, etc.

The savory herbs should be combined in a variety of dishes to find the most pleasing taste. With experimentation, the most delightful combinations can be achieved.

Do not forget that a single teaspoon of honey to a fairly large pot of greens or beans can enhance the flavor to an unusual degree.

Bold Print indicates items listed in the INDEX

IX. VEGETABLES

Scallions
(or Green Onions)

1 bunch scallions   3 T. water

Cut scallions in small pieces, using roots and tops. Sauté gently for 2–3 minutes. Cover and cook slowly for 10 minutes. Serve with **Cream Sauce**. Serves 1–2.

Scalloped Cabbage and Celery

3 c. chopped raw cabbage $\frac{1}{2}$ t. salt
$\frac{1}{2}$ c. chopped celery $\frac{1}{4}$ c. fine bread crumbs
$1\frac{1}{4}$ c. **Basic Cream Sauce**, thick

Cook celery, cabbage, and salt together for 10 minutes. Turn into floured baking dish. Pour **Cream Sauce** over cabbage and celery. Top with crumbs. Bake for 20 minutes at 350°. Serves 2–3.

String Beans I

Remove tips and stems and cook whole. Put $\frac{1}{4}$ cup water in bottom of pan, cover, cook until tender. Salt and herbs to taste. Variation: Serve with **Vegetarian Cream**.

Bold Print indicates items listed in the INDEX

String Beans II

1 lb. green beans, snapped
$1/4$ c. onions
$3/4$ t. **Curry Powder**
2 T. flour, whole grain

1 t. salt
$3/4$ c. water
1 T. lemon juice

Cook beans in a small amount of water until tender. While beans are cooking, place onions, **Curry Powder**, flour, and salt in a fry pan. Simmer until onions are tender. Add water and lemon juice. Cook gently for 10 minutes. Pour over drained beans and serve. Serves about 3.

Radishes in Cream

2 c. sliced red radishes
1 T. whole grain flour
$1/2$ c. **Soy Milk**

salt to taste
1 T. chopped parsley

Cook radishes in small amount of rapidly boiling, salted water about 1–2 minutes. (Radishes lose their color if overcooked.) Add the cream sauce made by cooking together the remaining ingredients for 5 minutes. Yield: 2 servings.

Kabobs

4 small onions, whole
2 carrots (2″ pieces)

3 radishes, turnips, **or** small potatoes

Hang on bamboo skewers or toothpicks and place in large kettle with $1/2$ cup water in bottom. Steam for 20 to 30 minutes until tender. About 2–3 servings.

Zucchini

Shred zucchini finely. Add about equal quantities of chopped onion. Place in deep kettle on medium heat. Makes own liquid for steaming. Serve with small amount of salt.

Green Beans in Casserole

green beans, cut, steamed
seasoned bread crumbs

Cashew Gravy or other gravy

Place cooked beans in casserole dish. Pour **Gravy** generously over beans and top with bread crumbs seasoned with onion powder and salt. Bake at 350° for 20 to 30 minutes.

Bold Print indicates items listed in the INDEX

IX. VEGETABLES

Squash En Casserole

2 qts. yellow crook neck squash, sliced in
    rounds
1 c. bell pepper, chopped
$1/4$ c. water

1 c. onion, chopped
$1/2$ c. brown flour
1–2 t. aromatic herbs
salt to taste

Place first four ingredients in a pot and sauté gently. The squash will release some fluid for steaming if they are young and tender. If needed, add some water. After about 10 minutes of steaming, cool, and mix in the flour and seasoning. Place in casserole, top with crumbs and sprinkle generously with paprika. Bake 1 hour at 350°. Serves 6–8. Variation: Add 1 cup **Golden Sauce** with the flour and seasoning.

Baked Summer Squash

4–8 medium crook neck squash, cut in
    two lengthwise, **or** 4″ chunks of zuc-
    chini

salt
food yeast
sliced garlic

Place squash on a flat baking sheet cut side up. Sprinkle with salt, food yeast, and sliced garlic. Bake at 350° for 45 to 60 minutes or until tender. Serve with a spatula. Good with a full menu of summer vegetables.

Stuffed Squash

summer squash, yellow or zucchini
onion, chopped
ground **Gluten or** Vegeburger

salt
garlic powder

Cut the squash, lengthwise in half for yellow, and in 6″ chunks for zucchini. Cut out the center seeded area with a paring knife. Place the seeded parts in a saucepan and steam gently for 10 minutes. At the same time, place the squash, cut side up in oven on shallow baking pans at 350° for 30 minutes. Put **Gluten**, chopped onion, salt, and garlic powder in the saucepan with the squash parts. Simmer gently about 5 minutes. Remove squash from oven, fill cavities with the gluten mixture. Return to oven for 30 minutes more. Serve hot.

Stuffed Peppers

5 medium bell peppers

4 c. **Spanish Rice**

Cut peppers in half, remove seeds and stems. Cook by steaming in a little water in a large kettle for about 10 minutes. Stuff each half with the rice mixture or leftover **Paella**. Place in a floured, covered baking dish at 350° for 30 minutes. Uncover and brown for 1 minute under broiler.

IX. VEGETABLES

Squash Tamale Bake

1 c. corn meal
3 c. tomatoes, quartered, packed **or**
   canned

2 c. squash, cubed
1 c. onion, chopped
2 t. salt

Place the ingredients together in a saucepan and stir until squash has released its juice well, and corn meal has thickened. After partly cooking, turn out into a baking dish. Bake at 350° for about 1 hour. Serve with **Sour Cream**, **Golden Sauce**, or **Pimiento Cream**.

Corn-On-The-Cob

Fill a large kettle with fresh, tender corn. Place about $1/2$ cup water in bottom. Boil vigorously until done (5–15 minutes, depending on maturity of corn). Do not overcook. Serve by itself or with **Pimiento Cream**, **Wheatonnaise**, or **Zero Dressing**.

Corn Stew

3 ears corn (yield 1–1$1/2$ c. whole
   kernels)
3 onions

3 green peppers, chopped
salt to taste
3 tomatoes, quartered

Simmer onions, tomatoes, and peppers gently for 5 minutes. Add corn and simmer for 5–10 minutes. Salt to taste.

Baked Corn

4 c. corn
enough water to blend

1 t. salt

Blend until smooth. Pour thinly into floured, flat pans. Bake 1–2 hours at 350° depending on thickness and water added, until slightly crusty on both sides. Score into squares with pizza cutter and serve hot with a metal spatula. Good cold.

Corn Kernels

Steam whole kernel corn in enough water to prevent scorching. When ready to serve stir in some chopped, canned pimiento or raw bell pepper. For variation, leave out pepper and sprinkle with parsley, fresh or dry.

Bold Print indicates items listed in the INDEX

IX. VEGETABLES

Eggplant Ideas

1. Slices of eggplant 1″ thick, salted, and baked for 1 hour until very soft. Chop garlic fine and sprinkle on top before baking.
2. Use cubes of eggplant on pizza.
3. Steam eggplant and onion together and serve with **Golden Sauce**.

Scalloped Potatoes

2 qts. potatoes
2 medium sized onions, chopped
$^3/_4$ c. cashews **or** pecans, optional

salt to taste
other seasonings as desired
2 c. water

Wash thoroughly, parboil and slice potatoes, jackets on. Arrange in a casserole alternating layers of potatoes and chopped onion, sprinkling each layer with salt. Blend the remaining ingredients. Pour mixture over potatoes and onion. Bake at 350° for $1^1/_4$ hours or until crust begins to form. Serves 6.

Mashed Potatoes

potatoes cooked in jackets
Soy or Nut Milk

salt

Use well cooked potatoes for mashing, about one for each serving. Mash potatoes, peeled or unpeeled, with enough **Soy or Nut Milk** to give a good consistency. Salt to taste. Variations: add raw finely chopped onion or scallions just before serving. Garnish with green onions or chopped parsley. Use **Sour Cream** or **Wheatonnaise** instead of **Soy or Nut Milk**.

Oven Potato Surprise

Spread cold **Mashed Potatoes** in a floured baking dish and make a depression in center. Place 2–3 cups of colorful, cooked, and seasoned vegetables in depression. Cover with **Mashed Potatoes** and broil at 450° for 10 to 20 minutes until light brown on peaks. Use green peas, chopped cabbage, any greens, carrots, etc. for the "surprise."

Hash-Brown Potatoes

4 c. potatoes, cooked in skins,
    chopped fine

2 T. unbleached white flour

Mix together and pour out into a baking dish. Bake 30 to 40 minutes at 350°. May need 1 minute under broiler to develop a brown crust on the peaks and edges.

Bold Print indicates items listed in the INDEX

Shredded Baked Potato

6 large potatoes, shredded
salt

$^1/_4$ c. lemon juice
pecan crumbs, optional

Place the shredded raw potatoes in a shallow baking dish. Pour the lemon juice over the potatoes. Salt lightly. Toss the potatoes a little with a fork to distribute the salt. Bake at 375° for 50 minutes until they are tender. Sprinkle with pecan crumbs and brown 1 minute under broiler. Serves 6–8.

Creamed Potatoes

cooked **Potatoes**, cubed

Holiday Gravy

Stir together and serve hot. Garnish with chopped mint or parsley.

Savory Potato Hash

3 c. diced, cold, boiled potatoes
$1^1/_2$ c. diced, cold entree, **or lentils,**
    or $^2/_3$ c. diced **Nuttose**
1 c. water, scant

3 T. diced onion
$^1/_4$ t. sage **or** marjoram
2 T. browned flour
salt to taste

Dextrinize the flour in a pan. Put the onion and sage into the pan. Add a small quantity of the water and stir smooth. Add the rest of the water and boil up. Salt to taste, and add the diced leftover entree to the gravy. Sprinkle diced potatoes with a little salt. Place in a baking dish and pour over them the hot mixture. Bake at 375° about 30 minutes to a light brown. Try this dish with **Turnips**, pumpkin, **Sweet Potatoes**, or **Butternut** instead of potatoes. Serves 4–5.

Bold Print indicates items listed in the INDEX

IX. VEGETABLES

Potato Curry

4 medium-sized potatoes
$1/4$ c. water
$1/2$ t. salt
$1/2$ t. garlic salt

$1/2$ t. **Nonirritating Curry or**
$1/4$ t. paprika
1 medium onion, chopped
1 green pepper, chopped

Boil potatoes in jackets and cut into $1/2''$ squares. Sauté onion, pepper, and seasonings in water and add potatoes. Simmer 5 minutes. Serves 4.

Thickened Tomatoes

1 qt. canned **or** ripe tomatoes with juice
1 t. salt

2–3 T. unbleached white flour

Season with favorite herbs if desired, or serve plain. Mix together and cook gently for about 10 minutes. Serve generously over **Grits**, **Rice**, or **Potatoes**. Use about $2/3$ cup for each serving. Serves 4–5.

Fresh Cucumber Relish

1 c. sliced, diced, or minced cucumber
$1/4$ c. lemon juice

$1/2$ t. salt
2 T. water

Place together in a jar and refrigerate, use as needed. Keeps 1 week.

Smothered Cucumbers

1–2 c. **Golden Sauce or Chee Sauce**   4–6 c. cucumbers

Cut cucumbers into cubes about $1/2''$ square and put in the sauce to simmer for about 20 minutes until tender. Serve as summer squash in a vegetable meal.

Georgia Gumbo

$2^1/2$ c. chopped ripe tomatoes
$1/4$ c. diced onion
$1^1/2$ c. cut okra

1 T. lemon juice
1 t. honey
1 t. salt, scant

Cook in covered pan on low heat about 25 minutes.

Bold Print indicates items listed in the INDEX

Baked Dressing

3 c. soaked bread cubes
$^1/_4$ c. diced onion
$^1/_2$ c. water **or** 1 c. tomatoes
$^1/_4$ c. brown flour

sage **and** marjoram
1 T. chopped parsley
salt to taste

Have the bread soaked in cold water until soft all the way through. Mix in all the ingredients lightly with a fork. Avoid breaking up the bread too much. Put into a floured baking dish, and bake until set and a nice brown. Serves 3–4.

Succotash

2 lbs. lima beans
2 c. whole kernel corn

1–2 c. **Holiday Gravy**
1 t. basil

Cook together until vegetables are done. Variation: For a one dish meal, add green peppers or okra and tomatoes. Add more or less gravy to make a sauce with it.

Baked Italian Eggplant

1 medium eggplant
1 c. **Tomato Sauce**

$^1/_2$ c. **Golden Sauce**

Slice the eggplant thinly and broil on each side 5–10 minutes. Alternate layers of eggplant, **Tomato Sauce**, and **Golden Sauce** in a floured casserole ending with **Golden Sauce**. Bake for 30 to 45 minutes at 350°. Serves 2.

Beets in Lemon Juice

$^1/_2$ c. water
$^1/_2$ c. Soyagen powder
2 t. honey
2 T. lemon juice

$4^1/_2$ c. shredded beets (raw) **or** 3 c.
   canned diced beets
salt to taste

Steam the shredded beets in 2 tablespoons water for 6 minutes. Mix water, Soyagen, honey, and salt in blender. Add the lemon juice. Heat slowly, stirring frequently until heated through. Mix with beets. Serve on **Dry Rice** or toast. Serves 4.

Bold Print indicates items listed in the INDEX

IX. VEGETABLES

Baked Okra in Tomatoes

Place whole, washed okra in a baking dish. Leave stems on. Pour in canned tomatoes to almost cover okra. Salt, and sprinkle dill seed or any other herb on top. Bake at 350° for 45 to 60 minutes. Leaving stems on prevents the development of the stringy character of okra.

Cucumber Gumbo

4 c. cucumbers, cubed
2 c. stewed tomatoes

salt, garlic, powder, and dill to
season

Simmer until tender.

Eggplant or Zucchini Stacks

large zucchini **or** peeled eggplant
tomato slices
onion slices

green pepper slices
cashew cheese

Slice zucchini **or** eggplant in $^3/_8''$ slices, allowing 2–4 slices per person. Soak eggplant in salted water $^1/_4$ hour, using $1^1/_2$ t. salt per quart water. This step may eliminate any bitter flavor of eggplant. Drain slices and place on oiled cookie sheet. Sprinkle with salt if not soaked. Place a slice of tomato next, then onion, then pepper, lightly sprinkling each slice with salt. Bake at 400° for 45 minutes. Remove and top each stack with cashew cheese. Bake additional 20 minutes. *nothing special*

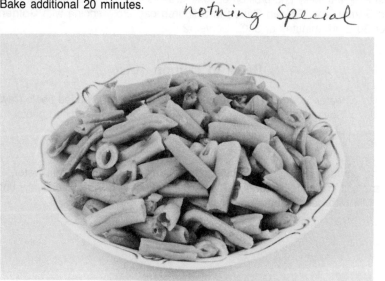

String Bean dish, page 142, 143

Creamed Carrots

cooked carrots
Nut Milk

salt to taste
onion

Place chopped carrots in blender with enough **Nut Milk** to barely turn over. Add $1/2$ onion to blender for each 4 cups of carrot mixture and blend until smooth. Salt to taste. Heat in oven before serving. Variation: use $1/2$ cup chopped, sauteed green onion per quart carrots.

Gajar

2 c. carrots, raw, chopped
2 c. **Soy or Nut Milk**
2 T. starch

2 T. honey
$1/2$ t. salt

Blend until smooth. Pour into a large skillet and gently boil 1 hour until most of the liquid has been evaporated and a thick paste remains. Pour out on a platter or pie plate to cool and thicken. Serves 4.

Dinner Carrots

4 c. carrots, cut into rounds
2 c. water, about enough to cover half the carrots
2 t. honey for each lemon used

2 T. starch
1 lemon, cut into very thin rounds
$1/4$ t. salt

Place starch and water in pan and bring to a boil, stirring constantly. Add other ingredients and gently boil until carrots are steamed tender, yet still crisp. Serves 6.

Breaded Carrots

8–10 whole carrots
Soy Milk

salt
Breading Meal

Scrub whole carrots and trim ends. Steam until done in a large kettle with a little water in bottom. Dip in **Soy Milk**, sprinkle with salt and roll in fine crumbs or **Breading Meal**. Lay on floured baking pan. Bake 20 minutes at 350° covered for first 15 minutes. Yield: 3–4 servings.

Turnip Cakes

Use the **Mashed Turnips** recipe. Add about 1 tablespoon flour to each cup of **Mashed Turnips**. Add grated onions or onion or garlic powder for seasoning if desired. Shape into patties, or drop by scoopfuls onto a floured baking dish. Bake at 450° for 20 minutes. Brown peaks lightly.

IX. VEGETABELS

Mashed Turnips or Rutabaga

4–6 c. turnips
1 onion

1 c. **Holiday Gravy or Basic Cream Sauce**

Steam turnips in little warm water until tender. Place in batches in the blender with onion and only sufficient gravy to blend until smooth. Mix well the several blender batches. Pour into shallow baking dish to keep warm in the oven. If desired may cover with crumbs and brown under flame. Serves 6–8.

Scalloped Turnips

4–8 sliced turnips
2 c. sliced onions

2–4 c. **Soy Milk**
1–2 t. salt

Parboil large, white turnips in a little water and slice into a baking dish in layers alternating with the sliced onions. Use about 1 cup of **Soy Milk** for 3 cups of turnips and onions. Add to **Soy Milk** 1 teaspoon salt for each 4 cups total. Pour salted **Soy Milk** over turnips and top with bread crumbs and bake for 1 hour at 350°.

Steamed Turnips

4–8 c. turnips
$^1/_2$ c. water

salt to taste

Place water and turnips in saucepan and boil about 20 minutes. Salt very lightly.

Baked Winter Squash

Cut hubbard, acorn, butternut, or any winter squash in 4″ squares. Place cut side down in a large flat pan with a little water in bottom. Bake at 350° until tender, 1–2 hours, and slightly browned on the cut edges. Serve with salt only. Delicious! Variation: Serve with **Coconut Gravy** or stuff with **Sweet Potato Casserole**.

Squash Delight

3 acorn squash
salt

$^1/_2$ c. light **Basic Cream Sauce**
$^1/_4$ c. corn syrup

Parboil whole squash 15 minutes. Peel and remove seeds. Cut squash into $^1/_2$″ wedges and put into medium-size, shallow baking dish. Sprinkle with salt. Combine **Sauce** and syrup. Pour over squash. Bake in 350° oven about 45 minutes basting occasionally. Then reset over to 400° and continue baking squash 15 minutes longer.

Bold Print indicates items listed in the INDEX

Sweet Potato Casserole

several well baked sweet potatoes   salt to taste
pecans, coarsely chopped, **or** peanuts

Peel and chop sweet potatoes in 2″ chunks, using 1 medium potato per serving. Add water and stir until there is a slightly thin potato juice, but many chunks remaining. Do not get juice too thin, nor leave chunks too large. Never add sugar to this sweet dish. Add $1/2$ cup nuts and $1/2$ teaspoon salt for each 4 cups of potato mixture. Bake 1 hour at 400°. May add orange peel or vanilla.

Baked Sweet Potatoes

Wash sweet potatoes of uniform size. Bake until tender at 400° about 45 to 60 minutes, depending on size. You can save time by cutting very large sweet potatoes in half cross-wise before baking. Cut crisscross gashes in the skin of the baked sweet potatoes on one side, then pinch them so that some of the soft inside pops up through the opening. Serve with **Gravy**. Save fuel by baking sweet potatoes when you oven-cook other food. If a moderate oven is called for, allow a little extra time for the sweet potatoes to bake.

Sweet Potato Balls

2 c. sweet potatoes, canned, or baked,   1 T. lemon juice
salted to taste   wheat germ **or** wheat bran

Mash sweet potatoes, salt, and lemon juice together. If too wet, add up to $1/2$ cup wheat bran. Make into balls the size of large walnuts. Sprinkle with wheat germ, using about $1/2$ teaspoon per ball. Bake 35 minutes at 375°. Serve alone or with a thin gravy.

Jerusalem Artichokes

1 lb. of artichokes $1/4$ c. water
salt to taste   chopped parsley

These vegetables are tubers. Put first three items in tightly covered pot. They may be steamed whole or sliced. If sliced, they will take about 15 to 20 minutes to get tender. Do not overcook as they may get mushy. Serve with favorite **Gravy**, chopped parsley, and salt. They are good steamed whole for about 30 minutes and then covered with **Golden Sauce**. Serves 4.

Bold Print indicates items listed in the INDEX

IX. VEGETABLES

Endive

> 5 endive (cut in half lengthwise)

Put $1/4$ cup water in bottom of pan, cover, steam until tender. Salt to taste.

Broccoli

Place frozen or fresh broccoli in pot with small amount of water. Steam until tender. Serve with lemon juice or **Vegetarian Cream**.

Watercress or Swiss Chard

> 1 bunch watercress **or** chard, chopped fine

Cook as **Broccoli** and serve with **Cream Sauce**.

Celery with Scallions

> 1 bunch scallions, chopped $1/4$ t. salt
> 2 stalks celery, sliced fine

Put $1/4$ cup water in bottom of pan. Bring to boil. Add vegetables, cover, cook until tender. Salt to taste.

Cauliflower

Place whole cauliflower, leaves on, stems down, in boiling, salted water ($1/2$ c. water, $1/4$ t. salt). Bring to a boil again, cover, steam until tender. Serve with **Basic Cream Sauce**.

Golden Cauliflower

> 4–6 c. steamed cauliflower   1–2 c. **Golden Sauce**

Place cauliflower in baking dish and sprinkle with salt if necessary. Pour **Golden Sauce** over the cauliflower and top with bread crumbs or chopped nuts. Brown at 400° for 10 to 20 minutes.

Bold Print indicates items listed in the INDEX

IX. VEGETABLES

Cabbage and Lemon Juice

Cut cabbage in wedges, leaving central core intact to hold wedges together. Place wedges in pot with a little water in bottom. Steam until tender (about 20 minutes). Drain, if much water is left. Use $1/4$ cup of the drain water and 2 tablespoons lemon juice mixed as a marinade to pour over cabbage. Serve with more of the hot marinade.

Cabbage

Chop cabbage desired size. Steam for about 5 minutes in small amount of water and season with salt.

Cabbage and Carrots

Chop cabbage finely. Chop carrots in strips and diagonal rings. Steam together in small amount of water until tender. Serve with **Chee Sauce** or **Golden Sauce**. Good served simply with lemon juice and salt.

Cabbagion

4 c. cabbage, finely shredded	2 T. water
$1/2$ t. salt	1 large onion, chopped

Heat all ingredients and cook gently until barely tender. Serves 3.

Garden Greens

greens, any type	lemon juice
onion, chopped	$1/4$ c. water
salt	

Fill a large kettle with the greens, such as turnips, collards, kale, dandelion, mustard, etc. Steam in the water and continue cooking until tender. The coarser greens require often an hour or more of cooking, whereas tender greens such as spinach will require only 5–10 minutes. Add the onion during the last 20 minutes if cooking time is long. Remove from kettle and drain in a colander. Add seasonings and chop finely. Serve plain, with lemon juice or **Tomato Gravy**.

Bold Print indicates items listed in the INDEX

IX. VEGETABLES

There is an ideal balance in the chemicals of the body. So precise is this balance that a very slight disturbance can result in prompt cessation of life. Consider the levels of sodium and potassium and the pH of the blood. The normal level of sodium in the blood ranges between 135–148 mEq/L. If the level goes as high as 160 or as low as 120 the person promptly dies. The potassium level is even more delicate. We usually have only 3.5 to 5.3 mEq/L, or about as much as would balance on a small pin head, in each quart of blood. If the level goes up to 6.5 or falls only as little as to 2.5 the person will suddenly die. Similarly, notice the very narrow range of the blood pH. The normal range is from 7.35 to 7.45. If the acidity of the blood falls only to a pH of 7.2 it is incompatible with life and the person dies. If the pH rises only to the level of 7.55 it is incompatible with life and the person dies.

Fortunately, we have many ways to keep these matters stabilized in the blood. If we are reasonably careful not to eat poisonous foods or foods that are so concentrated that the blood cannot keep itself within the narrow ranges required to be compatible with life, we can continue to live. There is, however, a great distance between "barely living" and having "optimum health." Recent advances in knowledge of nutrition give us understanding of many things that will help us to have more optimum functioning of both body and mind. We do not need to be "barely living." The use of all concentrated foods may endanger the body by imbalancing its biochemistries. Each imbalance must be adjusted, causing a tax on the body. Some of these adjustments cause accelerated aging and the body begins to wear out with such diseases as diabetes, heart and artery disease, cancer, arthritis, or mental illness. The concentrated foods include fats of all kinds, refined sugars and other refined carbohydrates, refined proteins such as meat substitutes and soy milk powder, wheat germ, nuts and seeds and their butters, food yeast, olives, and avocado. All of these should be taken quite sparingly and not too frequently during the month. Heavy proteins and oils have both been shown to be associated with a number of degenerative diseases, most notably cancer. As one grows older the need gradually diminishes for most nutrients, and less food should be taken in old age. A wide variety, however, should be maintained.

For all ages, oils should be measured by the teaspoon, not the tablespoon. Most nuts could be best numbered under half a dozen for a meal, and should be eaten at meals that do not contain other oils. The use of concentrated vitamin and mineral preparations is usually harmful to a greater or lesser degree. Fortunately they are generally not needed, and most people can simply forget about them. Food yeast has been reported to cause an elevation of blood uric acid.

Bold Print indicates items listed in the INDEX

X. SPROUTS AND SALADS

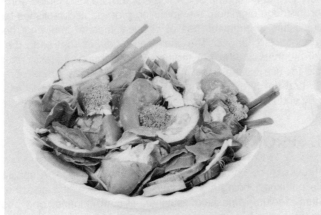

X. SPROUTS AND SALADS

ADVANTAGES OF SPROUTING

Seeds can be kept dry for many months or even years and are still suitable for sprouting. In preparing food for thorough digestion, the sprouting process accomplishes biologically what grinding accomplishes through the use of physical means, and what heating accomplishes through chemical changes. The chemical bondages formed in the seed for long term storage of nutrients are broken through the sprouting process, making them more easily available for use by the body. Additionally, there is the development of vitamins A, B, and C, and the formation of chlorophyl. Sprouting is said to increase the content of vitamins B_1 and B_2, niacin, pantothenic acid, pyridoxine, biotin, and folic acid.

SEEDS TO BE SPROUTED

Any seed that will grow can be sprouted in a jar, and used for food. A special favorite is **Alfalfa**. It is quite nutritious, being high in calcium and containing also the minerals magnesium, aluminum, sodium, potassium, sulphur, silicon, chlorine, and phosphorus. Alfalfa seed contain the entire B complex and are a good source of vitamins A, C, D, and E. To compliment the other good qualities, **Alfalfa Sprouts** are a delicious food. Radish seed, all the legumes especially including lentils, soybeans, and mung beans are suitable for sprouting. Lettuce, radishes, and similar plants that "go to seed" furnish good seeds for sprouting.

USES FOR SPROUTS

In winter, when greens are in short supply and are expensive in the market, **Sprouts** can be prepared in the kitchen for use at a very low price. One can do one's own organic gardening in the kitchen. This kind of gardening requires no weed killing and no mulching. With judicious planning **Sprouts** can always be ready for use.

Sprouts can be used separately with a little salad dressing such as **Wheatonnaise**, or used with other greens, tomatoes, celery, bell pepper, etc., as a tossed salad. Grated carrots tossed with **Sprouts** make a very fine salad. A good way to grate carrots is by putting them through a juicer and then mixing the juice back with the pulp to make a very fine grated salad. **Sprouts** may be added to soups at the moment of serving. A favorite way to serve a thick vegetable stew is to float a large handful of **Sprouts** on the top, and drop a dollop of **Wheatonnaise** on the mound.

Sprouts may be liquefied in tomato juice or **Nut Milk** in the blender to make a delicious and nutritious beverage, using a sprinkle of salt to prevent flatness. **Sprouts** may be sprinkled on potato or **Pumpkin Pie** for an unusual and crispy dessert. The use of **Sour Soy Cream** on top of the dessert makes a delightful blend of the sweet and sour. **Sprouts** may be mixed in breads, using them whole or ground in the blender. **Bean Sprouts** used as a main dish are very good as **Chow Mein**, **Burgers**, or as cooked **Lentil** or **Garbanzo Sprouts**. **Soybean Sprouts** are especially good cooked as a main dish. The cooking time is greatly reduced (to about 30 minutes) for difficult to cook beans such as **Garbanzos** and **Soybeans**.

METHOD

The simplest method for preparing **Sprouts** is by using a half gallon jar with a jar ring and a screen wire or piece of sterilized nylon hose. Three tablespoons of whole, unsprayed seed are placed in the half gallon jar with a generous quantity of water to soak overnight. The next morning the seeds are rinsed well, adding water through the wire screen or nylon. The jar is turned upside down to drain for a few seconds and then left with a kitchen towel covering the jar. Seeds sprout better in the dark. The seeds should be rinsed daily through the screen wire (more frequently in summer to prevent development of undesirable acids). Gently distribute the seeds around the sides of the jar by turning and shaking. The wet seed adhere to the jar wall. **Sprouts** are ready to harvest when $\frac{1}{4}$" to 1" long. Alfalfa seed can be allowed to develop up to 2" before they begin to get tough. Place the jar in the sun when leaves are ready, to develop the chlorophyl and vitamin A. Sprouting jars may get hot in the sun. Heat will kill the tender **Sprouts**. Watch carefully during sun exposure. Rinse **Sprouts** in water, using a large bowl to eliminate unfertile seed and hulls. Store **Sprouts** in a plastic bag in the refrigerator 1–2 weeks.

Sprouted Breakfast Cereal

1 c. sprouted wheat	4 c. boiling water
1 t. salt	1$\frac{1}{4}$ c. oatmeal

Stir oatmeal into boiling, salted water. Add sprouted wheat which has sprouts from $\frac{1}{4}$" to 1" in length. Harvest wheat sprouts immediately if any toughness begins to develop in either leaves or roots. Cook over low heat for 30 minutes. Serve as a breakfast cereal with **Nut Milk** or your favorite **Gravy**. It goes well with melon, sliced tomatoes or avocado. Serves 4.

Sprouted Lentils

Sprout 2 cups dry lentils. **Sprouts** are ready to use when $\frac{1}{2}$" to 1" long (3–5 days). In skillet, sauté until tender:

2 c. diced celery plus leaves	1$\frac{1}{4}$ t. salt
2 c. chopped onions	

Add the **Sprouted Lentils** and $\frac{1}{4}$ cup water. Toss with a fork and tenderize **Sprouts** 4–5 minutes. Then cover and let steam (low) for 15 to 20 minutes. A little garlic powder may be added just before serving. Serves 6–8.

Bold Print indicates items listed in the INDEX

X. SPROUTS AND SALADS

Sukiyaki

1 bunch green onions
1 large dry onion
$^1/_2$ c. sliced water chestnuts **or** peeled and
    diced radishes **or** turnips
$^3/_4$ c. water

$^1/_2$ lb. **Bean Sprouts**
1 c. sliced celery (slanting slices)
1 green pepper, cut in thin slices
seasoning salt, try celery salt
1 t. honey

Cut green onions in 1″ lengths, using most of the tops as well. Peel dry onion, cut in half, then slice in slanting slices. Sprinkle with kelp or vegetable seasoning salt. Heat in large heavy skillet along with water chestnuts, the **Bean Sprouts**, the water, and honey. Mix well and add the celery. Steam for 2–3 minutes. Add the pepper. Toss gently a time or two. Serve hot on rice. Scatter blanched and toasted almonds or toasted sesame seed over the top. Serves 4–6.

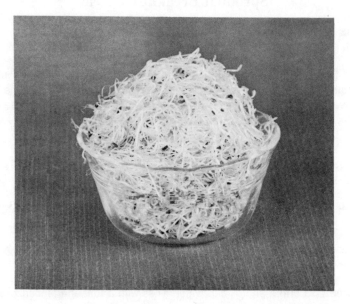

Bold Print indicates items listed in the INDEX

X. SPROUTS AND SALADS

VEGETABLE SALAD IDEAS

1. WHOLE VEGETABLE SALAD: Whole, well-developed vegetables are beautiful and delicious when served on individual salad plates with a sharp knife across the plate, garnished with a lovely flower or a sprig of parsley. Several vegetables are especially nice treated in this way: Tomatoes, sweet bell peppers, cucumbers, turnips, carrots, radishes, etc.

2. VEGETABLE PLATTER: Set a large center platter of whole vegetables of different sizes, shapes and colors, decorated with washed flowers, lettuce or other leaves, small branches of pine, etc. Set each place with a sharp knife such as a steak knife. The diners enjoy cutting their own vegetables and the saving in time is considerable.

3. LETTUCE BASKET: Pile high mounds of crisp lettuce leaves fresh from your garden in a nice, large basket lined with a pretty kitchen towel. Set one basket on each end of your table in easy reach. Encourage generous helpings of this low calorie food. It takes $3^1/_3$ heads of lettuce to make 100 calories. Serve the leaves with onion or garlic salt only, or with diluted lemon juice.

4. ALFALFA SPROUT SALAD: Place a bowl of **Alfalfa Sprouts** on a large platter and surround the bowl with various vegetables, either whole or cut. Shredded carrots piled around the bowl are beautiful. Lift first the **Sprouts** onto a plate, then some carrots, and top with **French Dressing** for a treat.

5. RAW SALAD: Any kind of mild, tender, edible leaf or flower may be eaten raw. In addition to the common greens, try watercress, spinach, dandelion, radish tops, chicory, lambs quarters, beet tops, parsley, comfrey blossoms, rose petals, geranium leaves and petals, turnip blossoms. Similarly, many vegetables and roots usually used cooked may be eaten raw: Try zucchini, yellow crookneck squash, Jerusalem artichokes, parsnips, turnips, young string beans, green peas. Furthermore, it is well to know that certain foods usually eaten only raw may be cooked: Try **Cucumber Gumbo** or cucumbers cubed in stews, radishes mixed with other cooked root vegetables or steamed alone, lettuce and comfrey mixed with turnip greens or other greens to make a milder flavored dish.

6. SALAD ENTREE: Generally, salads should not be rich or concentrated, since other articles of the menu are likely to have these qualities. However, if the rest of the meal is light, add nuts, seeds, unsweetened coconut shreads, food yeast, wheat germ, **Tofu**, or any cooked grain, **Pasta**, or legume. The salad may then be used as the **Main Dish** in the **Meal Planner**.

VEGETABLE SALADS AND COMBINATIONS

In all food preparation it is desirable to make individual dishes simple, and to serve few dishes at a meal. Care should be used that salads not become complex mixtures. Use one or two vegetables together, and serve attractively. Be artistic, and let each salad be beautiful.

VEGETABLE SALADS AND COMBINATIONS, continued

Radish Salad: Minced or shredded radishes and **Wheatonnaise**.

Cauliflower-Carrot Salad: Chopped cauliflower, shredded carrots, and **French Dressing**.

Shredded Cabbage: Well-shredded cabbage, served with a **Soy Cream**.

Tofu Salad: Shredded carrots, olives, **Soy Sour Cream**.

Potato Salad: Lay a wedge of tomato on each side of a salad plate with a scoop of **Potato Salad** in center. Olives or parsley to garnish.

Beet Salad: Ground, raw beets; ground, roasted peanuts; lemon juice.

Beet-Macaroni Salad: Cooked **Macaroni**, grated raw beets and chopped nuts. Moisten with a few drops of lemon juice. Serve generously, with soup and crackers as a full meal.

Sweet Potato Salad: Cube boiled or baked sweet potatoes. Add chopped nuts (1 tablespoon for each large potato used), celery, and **Wheatonnaise**. Use shredded turnips for celery as variation.

Carrot-Tofu Salad: Grated carrots, **Soy Cheese**, and **French Dressing**. Use as a main dish. Add a simple dessert, a special bread, or a few nuts for a complete meal.

Sliced Cucumbers

Have the cucumbers cold and crisp. Peel, if desired, and slice thinly. Just before serving, add a little **French Dressing** and chopped parsley, or they may be seasoned with lemon juice, salt, and a sprinkle of sugar.

Golden State Salad

Combine the following: 1 cup young carrots, 1 cup young turnips, 1 cup radishes, measured after being ground through a food chopper. Mix with **Wheatonnaise** and serve on a lettuce leaf or garnish with a liberal sprinkle of chopped parsley.

Raw Vegetable Dish

2 c. grated carrots	$1/4$ c. ground raw cashews, slightly
2 c. chopped celery **or** lettuce	toasted
$1/2$ c. shredded cabbage	1 t. minced onion
salt and mixed herbs as desired	2 t. lemon juice

Mix all ingredients together and chill. Serve with **Sandwiches** for a complete meal.

Golden Slaw

1 c. shredded carrots
1 c. shredded rutabaga
1 c. shredded cabbage

unsweetened shredded coconut
Soy Sour Cream

Toss the shredded vegetables together lightly. These vegetables make a delightful flavor combination. Place a tall slender server of unsweetened shredded coconut in the center of a large platter. Pile the shredded vegetables around the coconut. To serve, lift the shredded vegetables off with tongs and sprinkle top with some of the coconut and finish with a spoonful of **Soy Sour Cream**. Serves 6.

Tebula

An unusual salad that will surprise you!

4 tomatoes, chopped
2 peeled cucumbers, chopped
1 c. **Bulgar Wheat or Cream of Wheat**

$1/2$ c. lemon juice
$1/4$ c. Soyonnaise
salt

Place wheat in a bowl and cover with boiling water; set aside for 2 to 3 hours. Drain well. Toss soaked wheat with chopped vegetables, salt, and lemon juice. Green onions and parsley may be substituted for the vegetables as a variation.

"Cereal Tuna" Salad

$1/2$ green pepper
3 stalks celery
cold **Garbanzos**
3 c. cooked **Cream of Wheat or Rice**

$1/3$ c. Soyonnaise
salt, as desired
3 T. olives, chopped

Finely chop green pepper and celery. Drain **Garbanzos**. Mix all ingredients except olives. Place chopped olives on top of salad. Chill before serving. Makes 4–5 servings, about $2/3$ cup each. Serve with **Corn Fritos** for a complete meal.

Cole Slaw

6 c. shredded cabbage
Soyonnaise

$1/2$ c. coarsely chopped, salted peanuts

Combine cabbage, nuts, and enough Soyonnaise to coat lightly.

Bold Print indicates items listed in the INDEX

X. SPROUTS AND SALADS

FRUIT SALADS AND COMBINATIONS

Pineapple Salad: Pineapple slice, half of banana rolled in pineapple juice and dry bread crumbs. Top with **French Dressing**, **Coconut Cream**, or **Sour Cream**.

Rice Salad: Mix **Cooked Rice**, bananas (chopped, or whirled in blender with water), peanuts. Pour banana mixture over rice and nuts, or, if bananas are used chopped, serve with **Wheatonnaise**, **Soy Sour Cream**, or **Orange Sauce**.

Peach Salad: Combine cold **Cooked Rice**, sliced peaches, fruit juice dressing.

Fruit Salad: Drain canned peaches; combine with raw apples, raisins, or blueberries. Thicken peach juice with starch or agar and add to fruit. Top with **Soy Sour Cream** or Soyonnaise.

Ambrosia Salad: Dip sliced oranges into **Nut Cream**. Sprinkle with coconut.

Apple Salad: Combine diced apples, ground peanuts, lemon juice and Nut Cream.

Two-Fruit Salad: Combine equal parts of two fruits such as diced oranges, apples, pineapple, and bananas. Add lemon juice and a little honey to **Nut Milk** for dressing.

Use any leftover **Fruit Salad** in **Auf Lauf**.

Avocado with Fruit

avocado pears	seedless grapes **or** berries
Soy Cottage Cheese	orange wedges
French Dressing	plums
Corn Fritos	

Select ripe, small, avocado pears, peel them and cut in half. Put 2 tablespoons of **Soy Cottage Cheese** in each pear and stick any of the fruits all over the top. Add a little **French Dressing** and serve surrounded by crackers and more fruit as a garnish. Serve with a fruit sandwich as a complete meal.

Fresh Fruit and Sour Cream

3–4 qts. berries, any kind	1–2 c. **Sour Cream**
honey, if needed	

One of the nicest dinners possible on a Sabbath day is a huge bowl of fruit with a dish of **Sour Cream**. Use **Corn-on-the-Cob** or **Sesame Rice** as a main dish. Serve reheated **Oatmeal Buns**, **Corn Muffins**, or **Melba Toast**. Instead of berries one may serve sliced peaches, mangoes, apricots, or pears. Serves 10 to 15.

Waldorf Salad

2 c. diced tart apples	salt
1 c. sliced seedless grapes	$1/4$ c. sliced black walnuts
2 T. **Sour Cream**	3 T. lemon juice

Have the ingredients cold, then mix them together. Serve with **Melba Toast**. Yield: 4 small servings.

Diced Fruit Salad

Cut equal quantities of any two fruits such as orange, pineapple, banana, and ripe apple in small dice. Season with **Fruit Sauce**. A few ripe strawberries when in season are a good garnish, along with a sprig of mint.

Fruits and Nuts

1 c. diced oranges	chopped walnuts
1 c. diced bananas	

Mix the fruits, and moisten with **Fruit Sauce** or fruit juice. Dish up and sprinkle chopped walnuts over the top. Variation: Put two peeled, quartered oranges in blender and grind fine. Pour over sliced banana in a bowl. Top with nut crumbs.

Apple and Banana Salad

2 c. diced sweet apples	6 dates, chopped
1 large banana cut through lengthwise and sliced	**Fruit Sauce**

Mix the ingredients, and serve between 2 apple wedges placed in a circle on a salad plate.

Apple Salad

8 c. shredded apples	$1/2$ c. pecans, chopped
4 c. oranges, chopped fine **or** liquefied in blender	pinch of salt

While preparing shredded apples, apply some of the chopped oranges frequently to the apples to retard browning. The juice from the oranges is the only dressing needed. Toss with the pecans, or sprinkle them on top. Sprinkle faintly with salt if desired.

Bold Print indicates items listed in the INDEX

X. SPROUTS AND SALADS

Cranberry Relish

10 sweet apples
7 sweet oranges

1 lb. cranberries
pinch salt

Chop the apples fine. Peel 6 of the oranges, but leave the peel on one orange. Wash it well, scrubbing with a brush. Quarter all oranges to remove seed. Blend all oranges until fine in blender with salt. Put cranberries through coarse food chopper, or whirl lightly in blender with enough of the blended oranges to turn over in blender. Mix all ingredients. Chill and serve. May need to add honey if fruit not sweet. Serves 8.

Creamed Bananas

1 qt. **Nut Milk**
¼ c. tapioca

1–2 T. honey
vanilla, optional

Allow tapioca to soak in **Nut Milk** for 15 minutes. Boil for 5 minutes, stirring occasionally. Remove from fire. Add 2–3 sliced ripe bananas and mix well. Spoon over cereal or serve in fruit cups. Serves 4–5.

Herbs for Fruit Dishes

Almond Extract
Basil
Fennel Seed
Mint

Orange Peel
Sesame Seed
Vanilla

How to Separate Seeds from Small Fruit

Place the fruit in blender with enough water or fruit juice to cover fruit if fruit is not quite juicy. Whirl at lowest speed only enough to knock the seeds free from the fruit, but not enough to grind seeds. Some seeds are fragile and begin to break up with very little blending, such as watermelon seed. Ground seed often impart an undesirable flavor, but certain seeds should be ground up for the very purpose of imparting their distinctive flavor, such as wild cherry seeds. Pour from the blender into a wire strainer, the mesh selected for the size of the seed. Blackberry and ground wild cherry seed require an ordinary strainer. Watermelon requires a coarse mesh such as a vegetable colander or wire vegetable steamer. The resulting fruit pulp may be thickened for puddings or sauces according to the chart given in the section on **Dairy Product Substitutes**.

Bold Print indicates items listed in the INDEX

Asparagus Salad

fresh asparagus
romaine

watercress
French Dressing or Golden Sauce

Cook just the tender tips of the asparagus and chill them. Use the tender inner leaves of romaine and watercress which has had the stems removed. Make a bed of the greens on each salad plate. Place 4 asparagus tips on top of the greens. Spoon on the **French Dressing** or **Golden Sauce**.

Garbanzo Salad

4 c. **Cooked Garbanzos**, drained well
$^1/_2$ c. chopped onions
$^1/_2$ c. chopped celery **or** lettuce

$^1/_2$ c. chopped olives
garlic **and** onion salt
3 T. lemon juice

Mix lightly and serve as a main dish with **Soup** and crackers for full meal.

Lentil Salad

2 c. cooked lentils, **or** other beans
$^1/_2$ c. chopped green onions
fennel **or** tarragon

romaine lettuce
lemon juice

Chill the lentils and season to taste with the onions, lemon juice and herbs. Heap them in the center of a dish and garnish with crisp romaine lettuce.

Kidney Bean Salad

red kidney beans, cooked
minced green onions
chicory **or** lettuce, sliced

French Dressing
fresh tarragon, fennel, or dill

Chill the beans, and when ready to serve add the onions and bruised herb leaves. If these are not available, season the dressing with powdered tarragon or fennel. Toss the beans with the crisp lettuce or chicory and add the dressing. This is filling, and an excellent picnic food.

Bold Print indicates items listed in the INDEX

X. SPROUTS AND SALADS

<u>COOKED SALADS</u>

Potato Salad

cold, steamed potatoes in jackets
chopped or grated onion
chopped parsley to flavor

Garbanzos, about $1/2$ c. for each cup
   chopped potato
Soyonnaise

Chop the potatoes, skins on. Add onion, **Garbanzos**, and parsley. Sprinkle with salt and season with Soyonnaise or Nut Cream. To dish up, pile onto a platter, having the salad piled high and narrow, leaving the sides of the plate vacant for decorations. Garnish with lettuce or any raw vegetable.

Potato-Parsley Salad

6 c. cooked potatoes, diced
$1/2$ c. green or red pepper
2 T. lemon juice
$1/4$ c. chopped parsley

$1/4$ c. Soyonnaise
1 t. salt
$1/2$ c. onions, chopped fine

Mix ingredients and serve on crisp lettuce. Variation: Use canned pimiento, celery, or shredded carrots instead of bell pepper. Use spring onions with the tops instead of onion.

Hot Potato Salad

2 T. minced onion
1 t. parsley flakes
4 c. hot cooked potato cubes

1 c. **Sour Cream**
1 t. salt

Combine **Sour Cream**, salt, onion, and parsley flakes. Heat, if desired, but do not boil. Pour over hot potatoes and toss.

Italian Salad

2 c. cooked whole wheat **Macaroni**
$1/4$ c. chopped olives
1 c. shredded carrots

1 c. green peas
$1/4$ c. grated onion
Wheatonnaise as needed

The green peas may be used raw or cooked, as preferred. Mix all ingredients. Serve on a lettuce leaf. Serves 4.

Macaroni Salad

2 c. cooked and chilled **Macaroni**
1 c. chopped celery **or** bell pepper
4–6 green onions cut fine

$1/4$ c. sliced pimiento, optional
$1/4$ t. salt
2 T. Soyonnaise

Mix and serve. About 4 servings.

Cucumber Macaroni Salad

1 large cucumber
1 medium-sized bell pepper

1 medium-sized carrot, shredded
Wheatonnaise

Finely chop cucumber and bell pepper. Add shredded carrot and mix with enough cooked whole wheat **Macaroni** to serve 4–5 people. Add **Wheatonnaise**, onion powder, salt, and celery salt to taste, and a dash or two of lemon juice if desired. Refrigerate at least 30 minutes before serving. Serves 4–5.

Marinated Bean Salad

4 c. garbanzos
4 c. green beans
1 green pepper, finely chopped

1 onion, finely chopped
1 t. honey
3 T. lemon juice

Drain beans and place in bowl. Add green pepper and onion. Mix honey and lemon juice. Pour over beans. Salt to taste. Let stand several hours before serving. Serves 4.

Tomato Aspic

3 c. canned tomatoes
1 stalk celery with leaves
$1^1/_4$ t. salt
$^1/_4$ t. dill seed
1 t. paprika

3–4 T. agar flakes
1 c. tomato juice
$^1/_4$ c. lemon juice
1 c. celery, finely diced

Blend the first five ingredients until smooth. Cook the agar and tomato juice until agar is dissolved. Combine all ingredients and pour into single ring mold or small individual molds. Chill. Serve on beds of shredded lettuce or parsley topped with dots of **Wheatonnaise**. Serves about 4.

Turnip-Sweet Potato Salad

sweet potatoes, cubed
nuts, chopped
turnips, shredded

Basic Cream Sauce
Nut Cream
fresh mint

Use one sweet potato for each serving. Boil until quite tender but still holds together. Use 1 tablespoon chopped nuts and half of a 3″ turnip per serving. Use 1–4 tablespoons of thin **Basic Cream Sauce** per serving to moisten potato cubes well. Mix all ingredients. Top with Nut Cream which has been made with mint added. Garnish with sprigs of fresh mint, or sprinkle top with chopped mint.

Bold Print indicates items listed in the INDEX

X. SPROUTS AND SALADS

Scrambled Tofu Salad

1 c. chopped onion
2 c. tofu
2 T. chives
2 T. **Chicken Style Seasoning**

$^1/_2$ T. onion powder
1 t. yeast flakes
$^1/_4$ t. garlic
1 t. salt

Saute chopped onion in 2 tablespoons of water. Add the rest of the ingredients. Cook. Add **Soyonnaise** or dill weed dressing.

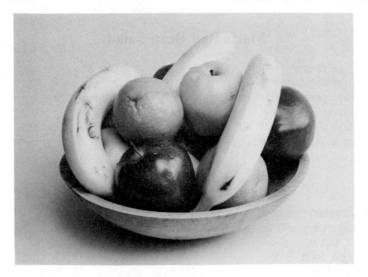

Fresh Fruit Platter

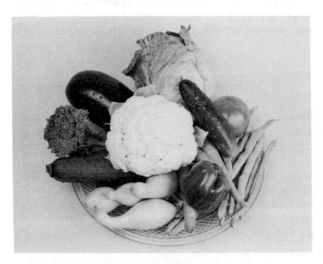

Vegetable Platter

XI. SANDWICHES

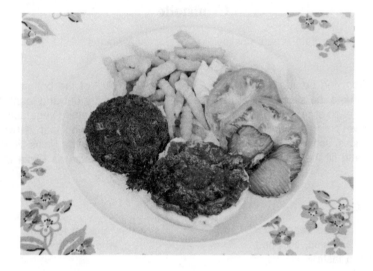

XI. SANDWICHES

Croustade

loaf whole grain bread, unsliced   seasonings
salt

Cut crusts from the bread. Cut loaf in $^3/_4$" slices to within $^3/_4$" of the bottom, leaving a solid base to hold the slices. Put loaf in the oven at 275° to dry out and toast. Sprinkle a little salt on each slice. Fill spaces between slices with fruit, creamed vegetables, **Chow Mein**, or leave plain. A giant **Croustade** may be made by cutting loaf in two to four lengthwise slices, scooping out the bread to make shallow beds in the slices. Slowly toast in the oven and fill the shallow beds with fillings mentioned, or use as **Pizza Crust**.

Bean Burgers

3 c. cooked beans   water, enough to blend
1 small onion, chopped $^1/_3$ c. whole grain flour
salt to taste

Stir ingredients together, mashing beans if desired, or leaving whole. Shape into burgers. Bake about 30 to 45 minutes at 350°. Serves 3–4.

Bold Print indicates items listed in the INDEX

Sloppy Joe

2 c. beans   1 onion, chopped fine
$^2/_3$ c. tomatoes **or** tomato juice, more
    or less

Place first 2 ingredients in blender and whirl to puree. Simmer the onion in barely enough water to cook until tender. Add to the puree. Salt to taste. Spread on toasted buns. Top with **Alfalfa Sprouts**. May sprinkle with chopped avocado or olives.

Pizza Sandwich

Spread slices of bread with **Catsup** or **Tomato Paste**. Add a generous layer of **Golden Sauce** or **Chee Sauce**. Dot with any of the following: **Agar Cheese**, **Tofu**, chopped olives, **Cooked Garbanzos**, braised onions and bell peppers, chunks of cooked eggplant, etc. Use any desired combination of the vegetables and cheese. Grill the sandwiches until edges are browned. Sprinkle with chopped olives.

Taco Sandwich

Place toasted bread in center of a plate and spread generously with chopped lettuce to make a bed. Sprinkle finely chopped tomato next, followed by onion slices. Finish off with a large spoonful of **Chili Beans**, and a topping of Soyannaise. Serve with **Corn Fritos**.

Bold Print indicates items listed in the INDEX

XI. SANDWICHES

SANDWICH FILLINGS AND SUGGESTIONS

1. Tomato blended with **Nut Butter**.
2. Mashed beans with **Tomato Paste**.
3. Dates, raisins, nuts, or bananas with **Emulsified Pecan Butter** or **Nut Cream**.
4. **Emulsified Nut Butter**, using half and half with blackstrap molasses or honey.
5. **Nut Butter** whipped with equal quantity of water.
6. Beans mashed with a little **Soyonnaise**. Onion slices if desired.
7. Avocado, onion, with **Wheatonnaise** or lemon juice.
8. Equal parts raw carrots ground or grated and **Emulsified Nut Butter** on one slice of the bread. With sliced tomato, delicious!
9. Peel tomatoes, slice thin, and serve with **Soyonnaise**. Add lettuce and thinly sliced onion as a variation, (or use only onion for an "ONION SANDWICH.")
10. Spread **Bean Puree** on bread, using lettuce and **Soyonnaise**.
11. Grind walnuts and dates through a mill. Season with lemon juice.
12. Slice cucumbers thin. Add grated onion and salt to taste. Make sandwich with cucumber, lettuce leaf, and **Nut Cream** or **Sour Cream**.
13. Chop celery very fine, and add chopped olives in the proportion of 2 parts celery to 1 part olives. Season with **Soyonnaise**.
14. $1/2$ cup finely chopped sweet pepper, 2 teaspoons chopped onion, 1 cup chopped ripe olives, with **Sour Cream**.
15. **Wheatonnaise** with 1 cup grated young carrot, 1 cup cooked peas, drained.
16. Grate carrots, chop peanuts fine, and mix together with **Nut Cream**.
17. Grind equal parts of nuts and raisins together and moisten with **Nut Cream**.
18. Slice cold loaf entree. Place on bread and spread with **Soyonnaise**. Top with **Alfalfa Sprouts**. A slice of tomato may be added.
19. Combine mashed banana and mashed avocado. Light sprinkle of salt.
20. Slice apples and combine with almond or cashew butter or any other **Nut Butter**.
21. Spread bread with **Soyonnaise**. Make sandwich with oatmeal patties and **Alfalfa Sprouts**.
22. Mash avocado, salt, and spread on bread.
23. Liquefy or puree **Garbanzos**. Add **Wheatonnaise** and spread on rolls. Place sprigs of crisp watercress between rolls.
24. Chop dates, nuts, and sunflower seed, together using twice as many dates. Grate into this $1/2$ teaspoon lemon rind. Spread **Nut Cream** on each slice of bread, spread with date mixture.
25. Mash ripe banana. Spread on bread. Slice papaya on banana and sprinkle over this crisp toasted nuts.
26. Grated carrot, chopped peanuts, and **Soyonnaise**. Mix lightly.
27. **Soy Cottage Cheese** and ripe olives or chopped tomato. Garlic powder if desired.
28. **Sesame Butter** with equal quantity of water or molasses beaten together to consistency of mashed potatoes.

Bold Print indicates items listed in the INDEX

29. **Soy Cottage Cheese**, sweetened with honey.
30. Special **Butters** such as apricot, apple, date.
31. **Soy Cottage Cheese** and pineapple.
32. **Hommus (Chick-Pea Spread)**. Puree 3 cups unsalted, cooked **Garbanzos** with the following in a blender until smooth: 1 clove garlic, $\frac{1}{2}$ cup **Tahini** (or $\frac{3}{4}$ cup sesame seed), 5 tablespoons lemon juice, 1 teaspoon salt. Use enough water in the blender to make the puree. Spread on crackers, **Melba Toast**, or bread.
33. **Peanut Meat** with tomato, onion slices, and **Soyonnaise**.

SANDWICH SPREADS

Mustard

$\frac{1}{2}$ c. water
$\frac{1}{4}$ c. unbleached white flour
2 t. paprika

$\frac{1}{2}$ t. salt
$\frac{1}{2}$ c. lemon juice
1 clove garlic

Cook these four items until thick. Return to blender and add 1 clove garlic and $\frac{1}{2}$ cup lemon juice. Whiz until smooth. Store in refrigerator up to 2 weeks.

Catsup

1 c. **Tomato Paste**
2 t. honey
1 t. salt

2 T. lemon juice
garlic or onion as desired

Whiz until smooth.

Bold Print indicates items listed in the INDEX

XI. SANDWICHES

THE ART OF LUNCHMAKING

Have a good lunch box that can be scalded and has holes for ventilation. Keep all lunch making supplies and equipment in one place near a convenient working surface. Let older children help in preparation of school lunches. Avoid a morning rush by having the lunch mainly prepared the evening before.

A good idea is to prepare a large batch of favorite sandwiches and freeze them. Wrap each in a cellophane bag, and date. Put one, still frozen, in the lunch box. It will thaw in 3–3½ hours. Leave out lettuce, tomatoes, and **Soyonnaise**. Send these in separate, individual containers to be added at the time of eating. Vary the type of bread used, but always use whole grains.

Do not be tempted to use very rich convenience desserts, as these desserts tend to promote an "all gone" feeling a few hours later. On special days send a special napkin, unusual fruit, a note, or a greeting card, rather than an unhealthful food.

PUT THESE IN THE THERMOS

1. **Soups**, creamed or chunky; always thick.
2. **Chowder**—corn, pea, vegetable.
3. Creamed dishes—peas, limas, corn, nut meats.
4. Hot **Fruit Sauce** to serve with **Zwieback**, toast, or cold whole grain such as rice, millet, etc.
5. Nutritious gravy to be served on **Brown Rice** or over a sandwich.

NOTE: Remember that foods kept at a high temperature for a long time lose some of their food value. Generally, only one food should be kept hot.

PACK THESE COLD FOODS IN COVERED CONTAINER

1. **Salads**—fruit, vegetable, potato, high protein such as peas and vegetables, or **Garbanzos** tossed with salad greens.
2. Fruit—fresh or canned.
3. Puddings—fruit tapioca, fruit whips, **Creamy Rice** with raisins, old-fashioned **Bread Pudding**.
4. Cobblers or simple fruit pies.
5. Olives.
6. Stuffed tomato or stuffed green pepper.

RAW FOODS TAKE THEIR PLACE IN THE LUNCH BOX

1. Must be clean and crisp and cool.
2. Vary the shapes for interest and attractiveness.
3. Wrap tightly or place in covered container.

Bold Print indicates items listed in the INDEX

4. These will be welcome—cabbage wedges, carrot strips or curls, cauliflowerets, celery curls or sticks, stuffed celery, green pepper strips, lettuce wedges, olives, tomatoes, radish roses, turnip dollars, any fruit in season. Remember to send along a sharp knife for paring.
5. Do not send a salt shaker. Teach children to relish crisp, raw vegetables and fruits without salt.

TIPS ON SANDWICH MAKING

1. Vary the seasonings and spread—parsley, onion, brewer's yeast, honey, lemon wedges.
2. Vary the bread as to kind and form—**Whole Wheat**, **Rye**, **Corn**, **Soy**, **Oat**, **Raisin**, date and **Nut**, **Pumpernickle**, **Muffins**, sandwich buns, **Zwieback**.
3. Vary the form of the sandwich—plain slices made into double-deckers or cut in various shapes, rolled up, made of brown or darker bread.
4. Spread the bread clear out to the edge.
5. Have the sandwich filling plentiful. Make it a good serving.
6. Crisp lettuce, watercress, parsley, **Sprouts**, and other greens make a tasty and nutritious addition to many sandwiches. However, usually they should not be added before lunch time. Send along in a separate wrapping.
7. Make sandwiches with neat edges.
8. Cut in sizes easy to handle and wrap securely.

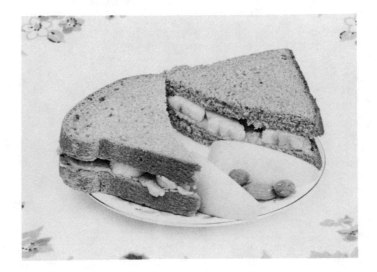

Bold Print indicates items listed in the INDEX

XI. SANDWICHES

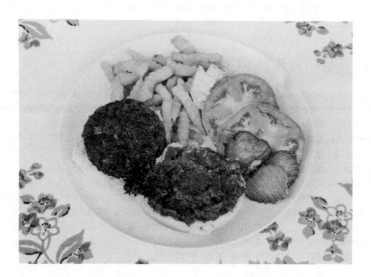

Bean Burger (page 172)

XII. MENUS

XII. MENUS

GENERAL PRINCIPLES

Planning the meal is often the most difficult part of preparing the family's food. Yet, it can be made simple by the use of a **Meal Planner,** and the knowledge of very few rules. By far the most important rule is that of eating a wide variety of vegetables, fruits, and whole grains.

Order is the first law of life. In no area is there a greater reward for attention to order than the family meals. The table should be one of the most neat and orderly areas in the house. No clutter should be allowed on the table. A small dish of greenery or a single flower will draw the mind to the Creator.

Orderliness in mealtimes and in gathering the family together as a unit will pay rich dividends. This is an important time for parents to shape the attitudes of their children while they enjoy the perfect fellowship of family love. No discord should be allowed at mealtimes, the family faithfully learning the discipline of self control in speaking only of pleasant subjects. There should be a strong family government to give the family members a sense of security.

There should be a set time and place for meals. An effort should be made to keep to the schedule. Remember that the digestive organs are on a **Circadian Rhythm.** They get prepared on time to receive food. Much energy is lost through irregularity. Many suffer fatigue or weakness for no other reason than an irregular schedule.

Similarly, menus should be made for each day and kept for a week or two. A quick review can be made to determine if the family is getting a proper variety. Excessive food or too many heavy foods can be spotted by the use of a **Meal Planner** such as the one given in this section.

TWO MEAL PLAN

Most people do better on two meals a day than on three. Careful attention to proper rest for the stomach lessens the likelihood of getting ulcers or gastritis. Since the digestive apparatus requires 5 *or more hours* to digest a meal, assimilate it, and get recharged for the next meal, it is taxing to the body's economy to crowd three meals into the stomach. No food should ever be eaten within several hours of going to bed, as recuperation from fatigue is seriously impaired if digestion is going on. The wisest plan is to take a large breakfast, a generous dinner, and no supper. Dinner can be taken in the mid-afternoon so that the appetite for supper is eliminated. If no evening food is taken, a good appetite for breakfast will gradually develop. Studies show that we need this meal more than any other. It gets all the biochemical systems supplied with raw materials. Make it a good one.

If a third meal is taken it should be light. Fruit and toast or plain crackers serve best as they are most promptly digested. Oils, nuts, and other fatty foods remain in the stomach much longer, and are unsuitable for supper.

LIQUID FOODS AND BEVERAGES

The digestion of solid foods is slowed if large quantities of liquids are taken with the meal. All the water must be absorbed before the solid portions can be brought in contact with concentrated digestants. It is well to promote the drinking of much water between meals, and to serve no beverage with meals. Encourage long chewing and mixing of foods with saliva. The starchy portions of the meal can be well along in digestion before leaving the stomach if small bites and long chewing are practiced. The pancreas will then have less work to do, promoting resistance to disease and health of that important organ. (Cancer of the pancreas has increased 400% in the past fifty years.)

Raw foods can be eaten in abundance if one feels thirsty during the meal. Gradually the inflammation of the stomach that calls for so much fluid will subside and the beverage or liquid food will not be missed. Raw fruits should not, however, follow a vegetable meal, nor should raw vegetables follow a fruit meal. To combine fruits and vegetables at the same meal can set up a war of competition for absorption sites and digestive processes. There is resultant mental dullness and loss of cheerfulness. Many experience headaches or some of the various evidences of poor digestion from a fruit-vegetable mixture.

RAW FRUITS OR VEGETABLES AT EVERY MEAL

To get a sufficient supply of vitamin C and to properly exercise the teeth and jaws, some food should be eaten raw at every meal. In some countries where great length of life is characteristic, such as Hunza, the people eat up to 80% of their food uncooked. Most fruits and vegetables can be eaten raw. Grains and legumes, however, should always be well cooked to make their nutrients available to the body and to detoxify certain properties that are injurious if taken uncooked. The cellulose framework of grains and legumes requires much cooking to break down the fibers to release the bound nutrients. The starch grains need to be converted to short chain dextrins. The action of heat and water will effect this conversion.

It is sometimes given as a reason for not serving uncooked food that the youth do not have a taste for it. A study done at the University of Nebraska showed a high percentage of students preferred fresh fruit and green salads, as many as 4 servings daily. An abundant supply of raw fruits and vegetables should be provided, at least one dish at each meal. The number of fruits or vegetables used in a single salad should, however, never exceed three, and one or two are better, to avoid **Complex Mixtures.**

Garnishing or decorating small salads is important. Wild summer flowers neatly arranged with alternate layers of green vegetables are pretty. In cold weather, designs cut from beets, turnips, radishes, or carrots add much interest to a salad. Daintily served dressings are among the most appetizing adjuncts of a meal. Don't forget the natural beauty of raw vegetables. Large platters or baskets of raw foods make lovely table decorations.

Bold Print indicates items listed in the INDEX

XII. MENUS

INTRODUCTION

BALANCE MENU BY THE DAY, NOT BY THE MEAL

In planning the menus it is not necessary to balance the nutrients at each meal. Studies show that we secrete into the bowel from the body stores a full complement of amino acids for the balanced absorption of the protein foods. By the day and by the week we should provide a wide variety. The body stores all food elements sufficiently long that if vitamin C is taken in the food daily and the other nutrients by the week, one can feel secure that one is adequately nourished.

Relative Acid and Base-Forming Quality
100 calorie portions

You may find it interesting to compare the qualities of certain foods in their ability to leave an acid or a base residue in the body. Generally, one may eat freely of the base-forming foods and sparingly of acid-forming foods.

ACID-FORMING		BASE-FORMING	
Oysters	30.0	Spinach	113.0
Haddock	12.0	Cucumber, fresh	45.5
Smelt	10.1	Celery	42.2
Chicken	10.0	Chard, Swiss	41.1
Egg, white	9.5	Lettuce	38.6
Halibut	7.8	Figs, dried	32.3
Whitefish	7.6	Tomato, fresh	24.5
Eggs, whole	7.5	Carrots	24.0
Egg, yolk	7.0	Olives	18.8
Beef, round, lean	6.7	Parsnips	18.2
Mackerel, fresh	6.7	Cabbage	18.0
Veal, breast, lean	6.7	Cauliflower	17.4
Salmon	5.4	Pineapple, fresh	15.7
Turkey	3.7	Orange Juice	14.4
Cracket wheat	3.3	Lemons	12.0
Shredded wheat	3.3	Apricots, fresh	11.0
Lamb, breast of	3.3	Radishes	9.8
Oatmeal	3.0	Potatoes	8.6
Barley, pearl	2.9	Raisins	6.8
Bread, whole wheat	2.7	Squash	6.1
Bread, white	2.7	Buttermilk	6.1
Rice	2.7	Apple, fresh	6.0
Mutton, chuck	2.0	Pears, fresh	5.6
Peas, green	1.2	Milk, whole	2.6

Bold Print indicates items listed in the INDEX

THE STAFF AND SPICE OF LIFE

See the section on breads to learn how important breads are in meal planning. Only in the most special of circumstances should breads be omitted from the menus.

EATING BETWEEN MEALS

There are some nutritionists who urge that one should eat between meals. Sometimes research is even cited to support the position that between meals eating is beneficial. In our practice, we have found that in all cases more than three meals daily are attended by some unwanted result. The benefits thought to require frequent feedings can be obtained by other, usually simple measures.

To eat more than three times daily draws the attention to food so frequently that life becomes little more than a round of wedging a few productive hours between great blocks of time used to satisfy the biologic needs. Little real good can be accomplished by such an individual and life becomes quite mediocre. As little time as possible should be spent on caring for the animal needs. Careful planning should lead one to derive the greatest benefit for humanity from each hour. The time spent in planning, preparing, eating, and cleaning up after numerous small meals amounts to a great wastage.

There are physiologic problems that arise from too frequent eating. In a study which we made to determine the level of toxic products that accumulate in the blood of individuals having a variety of meal patterns, it was found that more of these toxic products accumulate if many snacks are eaten, or if too many dishes are served at one meal. This study indicates that eating between meals promotes partial digestion with the production of aldehydes, amines, alcohols, esters, and other toxic substances from fermentation.

A study done on freshman high school students showed that students who ate between meals did not eat as well at regular meals as those not eating between meals. Sixty-nine per cent of the students reporting four or less "meals" a day were reported to eat well at meal time also. On the contrary, of those who ate ten or more times a day, only 10% were reported to eat well at mealtime. The rate of dental caries was proportionately associated with the frequency of between meal snacks. Even if the snacks are of milk, a food promoted as being good for the teeth, there is an increase in dental caries as the number of meals increases. An analysis of the various "meals" eaten showed that those students who ate 3 meals a day consumed a more balanced diet by far than those who were frequently snacking.

Those who are accustomed to eating at night often believe that they could not sleep without the evening meal. It is true that they may sleep the sleep of the drugged *with* the snack, but rest is not as good, and refreshment is impossible. There is less movement and better quality sleep in adults and children when a light, early supper is eaten, and nothing after. Restlessness and light sleep, often with unpleasant dreams, follows the "bedtime snack."

Bold Print indicates items listed in the INDEX

XII. MENUS

When new food is introduced into the stomach already containing partially digested food, the process of digestion of the original food is retarded. There follows inefficient digestion with putrefaction of foods and formation of toxins which get into the blood to dull the mind and destroy a good disposition. Symptoms of gas, heartburn, foul breath, disturbed sleep, irritability, and fatigue are experienced. A feeling of faintness is misinterpreted as hunger, but is actually digestive fatigue. Some hospitals are stopping the practice of between meal feedings because of these findings.

The normal stomach can empty after a usual meal in $3-4^1/_2$ hours. If a snack is taken after the regular meal has been finished, there is a burden placed on the digestive organs which cause the lining membranes to become weakened so that they cannot perform the functions of digestion, disinfecting and discharging with efficiency. The lining membranes of the nose and throat, which are close anatomical relatives of the stomach lining, sympathize with the stomach, and they, too, lose their efficiency in moistening, cleaning, warming, and disinfecting. Thus the person who eats between meals has his resistance to respiratory disease reduced.

Saliva is produced on a mealtime schedule for the person who is on a regular schedule. The salivary glands become filled with amylase to digest carbohydrates right on time to have greatest potency when food is expected. If food is taken ahead of time the preparation of amylase has not yet been made. If the meal is delayed an hour or two, much of the amylase is lost and digestion cannot be as efficient. Further, chewing gum or eating between meals keeps the saliva depleted of amylase causing poor digestion of the important foods of mealtime. The same unwanted results go on in the stomach and gallbladder. The gastric juices and bile show unwanted variations in their concentrations when there is constant digestion going on.

THE WATCHWORD IS VARIETY

Some attention should be given to the preferences of the family, to the colors used, and to the consistencies of foods. Meals are more satisfying if they contain a variety of colors, flavors, and consistencies, rather than being all yellow foods, all soft foods or all sweet flavors. The first rule in nutrition is variety. Foods chosen from among the vegetables, fruits, and whole grains will supply all needed elements for every member of the family except the breast feeding infant. Use vegetables generously, fruits freely, grains moderately, and nuts sparingly. The more concentrated the food, the less we should eat of it, as it is difficult for the body to handle concentrated foods. Furthermore, we need very little of a concentrated food to supply large quantities of nutrients. The surplus nutrients which have been eaten must be eliminated by the body, putting a strain on the biochemical systems.

TRAIN THE TASTE

More satisfying meals will be presented if each of the four primary flavors are included with each meal: sweet, sour, salt, and bland (used to supply the place of bitter which is a strong and unpleasant sensation to many). Train your taste to enjoy these flavors when they are delicate and not when they are pungent. Taking foods with strong or pungent flavors has been shown to promote overeating.

SECRETS OF PLANNING AND PREPARING A GOOD BREAKFAST

The Night Before:

1. Plan ahead what you wish to serve, and get things ready in advance.

   a. Plan interesting and varied menus.
   b. Prepare some new dishes.
   c. Repeat favorite foods, but don't get in a rut.
   d. Cook something with irresistable odor to stimulate morning appetites, such as **Melba Toast.**
   e. Introduce changes gradually.

2. Set an attractive table. If you have two sets of dishes, use them. Pick some wild flowers for the table.

3. Try the two meal plan, leaving off supper. Breakfast appetites will be hearty. Digestive problems will disappear. Children should be trained to the two meal plan at 1–3 years of age.

4. Get a good night's rest, going to bed and getting up on schedule every day of the week.

In The Morning:

1. Get all the family up in time to eat together. If someone must leave quite early, plan a special family breakfast on his at-home day.

2. Allow enough time to eat and enjoy it. Be prompt.

3. Cultivate cheerfulness without overdoing it.

4. Allow individual choice of kind and amount of low calorie and raw foods. Consider serving individual portions of concentrated or high calorie foods to avoid overeating on them.

5. Avoid sameness from day to day.

Bold Print indicates items listed in the INDEX

XII. MENUS

MEAL PLANNER
_____

MEAL PLANNER

	Main Dish (Good in Protein and B-vitamins)	Second Dish (May be Cooked or Raw)	Raw Dish (Good in vitamin C)	Whole Grain Bread (Select one, any kind)	Spread, Nuts, Olives, or Avocado
SUNDAY **Breakfast** **Dinner**					
MONDAY **Breakfast** **Dinner**					
TUESDAY **Breakfast** **Dinner**					
WEDNESDAY **Breakfast** **Dinner**					
THURSDAY **Breakfast** **Dinner**					
FRIDAY **Breakfast** **Dinner**					
SABBATH **Breakfast** **Dinner**					

Copy this **Meal Planner.** Use it daily in your planning. Select **Main Dishes** from the list that follows this **Meal Planner.** Select items for the fifth column from the list of **Spreads and Side Dishes.** If you are faithful in using a **Meal Planner,** you will not get nutritional deficiencies or excesses. The main dish should provide 200–300 calories per serving. Each of the other columns should provide 50–100 calories, depending on the needs of the person.

XII. MENUS

Main Dishes

SHOULD BE GOOD SOURCES OF PROTEIN AND B-VITAMINS
SHOULD SUPPLY 200–300 CALORIES PER SERVING

Legumes
Beans
Peas
Peanuts
Lentils
Garbanzos

Grains
Corn
Rice
Wheat
Oats
Buckwheat
Millet
Rye
Barley
Triticale
Popcorn

Certain Tubers
Potatoes, sweet and white
Carrots
Turnips
Rutabagas
Jerusalem artichokes
Parsnips

Seeds
Nuts
Sunflower
Sesame
Pumpkin

Certain Vegetables
(Too low in calories to
provide 200–300. Other
features excellent.)
Asparagus
Broccoli
Brussel sprouts
Spinach
Collards
Turnip greens

Other Foods
Winter squash
Pumpkins
Okra

Spreads and Side Dishes

USE 1–2 TEASPOONS OF THE CONCENTRATED FOODS AND UP TO
¼ CUP OF THE LESS CONCENTRATED ITEMS

Nuts and Nut Butters
Almonds
Walnuts
Peanuts
Coconut
Filberts
Pine
Cashews
Other

Spreads
Wheatonnaise
Soy Sour Cream
Butters (fruit or
cereal)

Bland Fruits
Olives, 4–6
Avocado, ¼–⅓

Seeds
Sunflower
Pumpkin
Sesame

Gravies and Sauces
Cream Sauce
Nut Gravies
Brown Gravy

Bold Print indicates items listed in the INDEX

XII. MENUS

SIMPLICITY

One of the great principles of life is that of simplicity. Every aspect of life can reflect this profound feature. The lifestyle, from possessions to the manners taught to one's children, can reveal this godlike quality. Simplicity does not imply carelessness or halfheartedness. Both of these characteristics reveal weakness of the fabric of the personality. To make a simple lifestyle the pattern of the life requires dedication, as the tendency of modern life is always toward more sophistication, more gloss and veneer.

In the kitchen, one's possessions and equipment should not exceed the storage space available. A scrupulously clean kitchen, with every article put away and all decks cleared, will go far toward making a happy home. The disordered mind manifested by unfinished work in the kitchen leads to querulousness and irritation, and a sense of dissatisfaction with home. Every woman should consider it a mark of her genius to keep the home neat. Children should be taught as early as possible to cook and to clean the kitchen. Habits of orderliness should be carefully instilled from the earliest experience. Such a child, having been taught to love well-disciplined work will have his happiness and mental balance assured.

Simplicity in regard to food includes not only the number of dishes served, and the complexity of each dish served, but the concentration of each food item used. If many highly concentrated foods are used in a single meal the digestive organs will be taxed to properly digest and dispose of the heavy nutrients without injury to the delicate mechanisms. It is within the experience of all to have the inside of the mouth pucker when a substance of high concentration is held in the mouth. The concentrated substance actually alters the chemical makeup of the lining cells of the mouth. The same sort of process occurs in the stomach and inside the bloodstream if concentrated nutrients are introduced into them. Oils are very concentrated food substances. The stomach and intestines have several special mechanisms for handling them. This is a very elaborate feedback arrangement to insure that only a small quantity is allowed into the duodenum from the stomach. So efficient is this mechanism that only 10 grams of fat (about 2 teaspoons) will be permitted to leave the stomach in one hour. Therefore a lot of fat mixed in a meal causes stagnation of food in the stomach. Fermentation is more likely to occur with stagnation. Toxic products of fermentation make the blood impure.

Oils are handled by the digestive tract in a different manner from other nutrients, being emulsified in the duodenum and taken up mainly in the lymphatic vessels, not in the blood vessels. The lymphatic vessels form a one-way system from the intestines to a large blood vessel in the chest where the material picked up by the lymphatic vessels is introduced into the blood stream. The fluid in the lymphatic vessels is milky after a meal because of all the emulsified fat from the last meal. The more fat in the meal the more milky the blood plasma becomes. Most people are frightened when they see the color of their blood plasma when a sample is drawn just after a meal containing the usual American fat allotment. Fat in the blood plasma causes the blood to clot more easily. If

Bold Print indicates items listed in the INDEX

XII. MENUS

the blood clots very readily, clots form inside the blood vessels, and one is in trouble. Not only do clots form more readily (a function performed by the plasma itself) but the red blood cells also stick together in small clusters when a meal containing fats of any kind has been eaten. These clusters of blood cells are not clots. Yet they will plug up small capillaries. The more fat eaten, the more of these little red blood cell clusters can be found in the blood and the greater the danger of damage to vital areas such as the brain, kidneys, pancreas, adrenals, and other very highly developed blood vessel fields.

Of course, all are aware that the incidence of heart attacks is higher in countries consuming more of their calories in the form of fats. Everyone is not, however, aware that cancer is also higher in countries consuming more of their calories from fats. In the last few years polyunsaturated fats have come under condemnation because of this relationship. Any concentrated nutrient is potentially harmful if taken in quantity other than sparingly. How important that all rich, or concentrated, foods be limited. Reason tells one that this is true. We need not wait until medical science has reported toxicity from some concentrated food to begin a reasonable program of eating. Custom is not a reliable guide for planning the food one will eat. A serious evaluation of each food used in the menu is the only way to arrive at a safe and sensible dietary.

It is necessary that humans obtain a wide variety of food in order to insure a balance of nutrients, to store the needed trace elements, and to provide a pleasing variety. It is not necessary to have the most expensive foods, however, in order to be well nourished. The grains, with fruits, nuts, and vegetables contain all the nutritive properties necessary to make good blood. It is not necessary, however, to have all of these food groups on the menu at each meal. Generally speaking, a well balanced breakfast consists of whole grains and fruits, and a well balanced dinner consists of whole grains and vegetables. Nuts may or may not be added to either meal. Nuts should be used sparingly. The number of dishes should be from two to four. For routine fare, and when one has especially heavy responsibilities, or when there are family crises, the more simple the menus the better. The use of fruits and grains only for a few days may be advantageous. All food elements need not be supplied at each meal, but, rather, the meals should be balanced over a period of a week, month or year. If circumstances demand it, several days of fruit meals may be used without doing damage to the general nutrition. For those whose work is sedentary or involves heavy brain work such a course will be especially helpful.

In many cases of sickness a fast for a meal or two may be of great relief. If this is followed by a few days of a fruit diet one may be restored to health. Those who are weary and nervous from constant application to confining labor will find that a visit to the country where a simple, carefree life may be obtained, coming in close contact with nature, and sensing the beauty of the created flora and fauna will be more beneficial than any other agency in bringing recovery.

Bold Print indicates items listed in the INDEX

XII. MENUS

SAMPLE MENUS

MEAL PLANNER

Low Cholesterol Diet

Day	Main Dish (Good in Protein and B-vitamins)	Second Dish	Raw Dish (Good in vitamin C)	Whole Grain Bread	Spread, Nuts, Olives, or Avocado
SUNDAY Breakfast	Sesame Rice		Fresh Fruit and Soy Sour Cream	Zwieback	Soy Sour Cream / Chee Sauce / Cashew Pimiento Cheese
Dinner	Bean Pot	Baked Summer Squash	Lettuce Basket	Pumpernickel	
MONDAY Breakfast	Grits and Peanut Gravy	Fresh Applesauce	grapefruit	crackers	Peanut Butter
Dinner	Soy Patties	Jerusalem Artichokes	Alfalfa Sprout Salad	Whole Wheat Bread	Almond Gravy
TUESDAY Breakfast	All Bran	Orange Sauce	Apple Salad	crackers	Apple Butter
Dinner	Chili Grits	Garden Greens	Golden Slaw	Swedish Almond Braid	Tomato Gravy
WEDNESDAY Breakfast	Cream of Rye	Sautéed Breakfast Apples	Waldorf Salad	Melba Toast	Apricot Butter
Dinner	Patties	Radishes in Cream	Beet-Macaroni Salad	crackers	
THURSDAY Breakfast	Maranola	Creamed Bananas	grapefruit	Rye Bread	Carob Sauce
Dinner	Soy Cheese Balls	Squash Delight	Shredded Cabbage	Corn Muffins	gravy
FRIDAY Breakfast	Baked Grits		Two Fruit Salad	Whole Wheat Toast	Soyannaise on Grits
Dinner	Hoppin' John	Cabbage and Lemon	Tofu Salad	Whole Wheat Bread	Basic Cream Sauce
SABBATH Breakfast	Cream of Wheat	Fruit Sauce	Diced Fruit Salad	Wheat Gems	Apple Butter
Dinner	Hommus Tahini (use as spread)	Golden Cauliflower	Tebula	Zwieback for Open Face Sandwiches	Nut Dressing

Bold Print indicates items listed in the INDEX

SAMPLE MENUS

MEAL PLANNER — Low Cholesterol Diet

	Main Dish (Good in Protein and B-vitamins)	Second dish	Raw Dish (Good in vitamin C)	Whole Grain Bread	Spread, Nuts, Olives, or Avocado
SUNDAY Breakfast	Corn Dodgers	Blackberry Sauce	wild plums	Whole Wheat Toast	Pear Butter / lemon juice
Dinner	Arroz con Pollo	Squash En Casserole	Vegetable Platter		
MONDAY Breakfast	Corn Waffles	Stewed Apricots	tangerine	Corn Waffles	Emulsified Cashew Butter
Dinner	Sprouted Lentils	Kabobs	Shredded Cabbage	Zwieback	
TUESDAY Breakfast	Rice Fritters	Prune Whip	strawberries	Corn Muffins	Basic Cream Sauce
Dinner	Blackeyed Peas, East Indian Style	Scalloped Cabbage and Celery	"Cereal Tuna" Salad	Whole Wheat Bread	Cashew Gravy
WEDNESDAY Breakfast	Apple Icing Bread	Cranberry Relish	orange		Cocopeanut Cream
Dinner	baked potatoes	String Beans	Vegetable Platter	Soy Bread	Pimiento Cream
THURSDAY Breakfast	Corn Meal Mush	Applesauce	plums	Whole Wheat Crackers	Cashew Gravy
Dinner	Chinese Pepper Steak	Scalloped Turnips	Golden State Salad	Zwieback	Nut Dressing
FRIDAY Breakfast	Grapenuts	Orange Sauce	Apple Salad	Pumpernickel Toast	Apple Butter / lemon juice
Dinner	Sukiyaki	Rice	Sliced Cucumbers	Gem Dandies	
SABBATH Breakfast	Scrambled Tofu	Grits	Cantaloupe	Zwieback	Soy Sour Cream
Dinner	Holiday Roast	Zucchini	Raw Salad	Corn Bread	Nut Gravy

Bold Print indicates items listed in the INDEX

XII. MENUS

192

SAMPLE MENUS

MEAL PLANNER

Hypoglycemia Diet	Main Dish (Good in Protein and B-vitamins)	Second Dish	Raw Dish (Good in vitamin C)	Whole Grain Bread	Hypoglycemia Diet — Spread, Nuts, Olives, or Avocado
SUNDAY Breakfast	**Fruited Oats**		**Blackberry Sauce**	**Corn Bread**	pumpkin seed (1 oz.)
Dinner	**Scalloped Potatoes**	asparagus	carrot strips	**Whole Wheat Bread**	olives (4–6)
MONDAY Breakfast	**Baked Grits Squares**	**Pear Butter**	grapes	**Whole Wheat Toast**	**Almond Gravy**
Dinner	**Chop Suey**	**Brown Rice**	**Cole Slaw**	**Corn Fritos**	**Soy Sour Cream**
TUESDAY Breakfast	**Buckwheat-Rice Cereal**	stewed apricots	orange	**Melba Toast**	almond milk
Dinner	**Corn Tamale Pie**	English peas	sliced tomatoes	**Hush Puppies**	gravy
WEDNESDAY Breakfast	**Corn Meal Soufflé**	**Sautéed Apples**	pear	**Tortillas**	olives
Dinner	boiled potatoes		onion slices	**Whole Wheat Bread**	
THURSDAY Breakfast	**Corn Oat Waffles**	stewed apricots	plums (2)		emulsified pecan butter
Dinner	lentils		shredded carrots	**Carrot Corn Bread**	olives (4–6)
FRIDAY Breakfast	**Corn Meal Mush**	**Applesauce**	orange	**Melba Toast**	pecans
Dinner	**Oat Burgers**	sliced tomatoes/onions	**Alfalfa Sprouts**	burger buns	**Mustard & Catsup**
SABBATH Breakfast	**Auf Lauf**	thickened fruit juice	peaches	**Corn Bread**	**Nut Milk**
Dinner	**Tofu, Oven Method**	**Zucchini Squash**	lettuce wedges	**Melba Toast**	gravy

Bold Print indicates items listed in the INDEX

MEAL PLANNER

Hypoglycemia Diet

Day / Meal	Main Dish (Good in Protein and B-vitamins)	Second Dish	Raw Dish (Good in vitamin C)	Whole Grain Bread	Spread, Nuts Olives, or Avocado
SUNDAY					
Breakfast	oatmeal		**Fruit Sauce**	**Melba Toast**	almonds, toasted
Dinner	**Spanish Rice**		sliced tomatoes	**Corn Dodgers**	olives (4–6)
MONDAY					
Breakfast	**Rice Pudding**	stewed baked pears	seedless grapes	**Corn Fritos**	**Nut Milk**
Dinner	dry beans	summer squash	celery sticks	**Oatmeal Buns**	**Sesame Butter**
TUESDAY					
Breakfast	**French Toast**	**Applesauce or** strawberries	tart apple		pecan butter
Dinner	**Dry Rice**	bean soup	carrot strips	**Zwieback**	avocado
WEDNESDAY					
Breakfast	**Millet**		**Fruit Sauce**	**Melba Toast**	cashews
Dinner	**Split Pea Soup**	**Butternut Squash**	cucumber/lemon juice	**Croutons**	Pumpkin seed (1 oz.)
THURSDAY					
Breakfast	baked oatmeal	stewed peaches	blackberries	**Popcorn**	carob-nut milk
Dinner	**Garbanzos**	corn and okra	lettuce	**Baked Corn**	olives (4–6)
FRIDAY					
Breakfast	**Granola**	**Fruit Sauce**	cherries	rye toast	**Sesame Butter**
Dinner	**Soy Loaf**	**Zucchini**	tomato	**Oatmeal Buns**	**Gravy**
SABBATH					
Breakfast	**Grits**		apples	**Melba Toast**	peanuts, toasted
Dinner	**Bean Puree** over split **Corn Muffins**	brussel sprouts	bell peppers	**Corn Muffins**	**French Dressing**

Bold Print indicates items listed in the INDEX

XII. MENUS

SAMPLE MENUS

MEAL PLANNER

Low Protein	Main Dish (Good in Protein and B-vitamins)	Second Dish	Raw Dish (Good in vitamin C)	Whole Grain Bread	Low Protein — Spread, Nuts, Olives, or Avocado
SUNDAY Breakfast	Lentil Porridge		melons	Doughnuts	Carob Sauce
SUNDAY Dinner	Noodles with Asparagus	Cauliflower	Radish Salad	Whole Wheat Bread	French Dressing
MONDAY Breakfast	French Toast	Chestnut Chutney	apple	Corn Muffins	honey
MONDAY Dinner	Tomato and Okra Pilau	String Beans	Cole Slaw	Oatmeal Buns	
TUESDAY Breakfast	Soy Waffles	Queen Fruit Sauce	strawberries	Soy Waffles	emulsified almond butter
TUESDAY Dinner	Bread Dressing	Thickened Tomatoes	Raw Vegetable Dish	Whole Wheat Bread	lemon juice
WEDNESDAY Breakfast	Hominy Grits	Sauteed Breakfast Apples	oranges	Melba Toast	
WEDNESDAY Dinner	Macaroni with Green Peppers	Endive	Cauliflower-Carrot Salad	Aerated Oatmeal Gems	French Dressing
THURSDAY Breakfast	Fruited Oats		grapefruit	Whole Wheat Toast	Nut Milk
THURSDAY Dinner	Millet Loaf	Baked Eggplant	Lettuce Basket	Barley Cakes	Cashew Pimiento Cheese
FRIDAY Breakfast	Buckwheat Rice Cereal	Raisin Sauce	apple	Baked Millet	
FRIDAY Dinner	Chili Grits	Broccoli	Vegetable Platter	Whole Wheat Bread	lemon wedges
SABBATH Breakfast	Corn Waffles	Applesauce	blackberries	Corn Waffles	emulsified sesame butter
SABBATH Dinner	Creole	Baked Okra in Tomatoes	Carrot-Tofu Salad	Corn Muffins	French Dressing

Bold Print indicates items listed in the INDEX

SAMPLE MENUS

MEAL PLANNER

Low Protein	Main Dish (Good in Protein and B-vitamins)	Second Dish	Raw Dish (Good in vitamin C)	Whole Grain Bread	Low Protein — Spread, Nuts, Olives, or Avocado
SUNDAY **Breakfast**	**Fruit Pie**	**Tropical Cereal Sauce**	**Rice Salad**	**Whole Wheat Toast**	**Apple Butter**
Dinner	**Macaroni Chee**	**Scallions**	bell peppers		olives
MONDAY **Breakfast**	**Swedish Farina**	**Queen Fruit Sauce**	grapes	**Popovers**	**Carob-Tahini Butter**
Dinner	**Nuttose**	**Calsoup**	sliced tomatoes	**Whole Wheat Bread**	lemon juice
TUESDAY **Breakfast**	**French Toast**	**Fruit Juice Sauce**	pear		emulsified pecan butter
Dinner	**Noodles** with Asparagus	**Baked Okra in Tomatoes**	**Lettuce Basket**		avocado
WEDNESDAY **Breakfast**	**Berry Pie**	**Swiss Chard**	**Peach Salad**	**Rye Bread**	**Vanilla Sauce**
Dinner	**Chow Mein** and Dry Rice		**Whole Vegetable Salad**	**Corn Fritos**	**Soy Sour Cream**
THURSDAY **Breakfast**	**Apple Icing Bread**	**Fruit Sauce**	apple	**Popcorn**	toasted nuts
Dinner	**Okra Patties**	**Cream of Cabbage Soup**	tomato wedges	**Whole Wheat Bread**	lemon juice
FRIDAY **Breakfast**	**Corn Oat Waffles**	**Banana Cereal Sauce**	persimmons	**Corn Oat Waffles**	emulsified tahini
Dinner	**Corn Tamale Pie**	**Celery with Scallions**	**Beet Salad**		**Lemon and Onion Dressing**
SABBATH **Breakfast**	**Millet**	**Cabbagion**	**Ambrosia Salad**	**Whole Wheat Toast**	**Nut Dressing on Millet**
Dinner	**Lasagna**		**Potato Salad**		olives

Bold Print indicates items listed in the INDEX

XII. MENUS

SAMPLE MENUS

MEAL PLANNER

Regular Diet		Main Dish (Good in Protein and B-vitamins)	Second Dish	Raw Dish (Good in vitamin C)	Whole Grain Bread	Spread, Nuts, Olives, or Avocado (Regular Diet)
SUNDAY	Breakfast	oatmeal	raisins on oatmeal	**Applesauce**	**Corn Bread** with honey	toasted peanuts
	Dinner	**Chili Beans**	(**Main Dish** has 2 veg.)	**Cole Slaw**	**Zwieback**	olives (4–6)
MONDAY	Breakfast	**Auf Lauf**	thickened fruit juice	orange	**Corn Fritters**	**Nut Cream**
	Dinner	**Oat Burgers**	baked zucchini chunks	sliced tomatoes & onion	**Whole Wheat Buns**	**Mustard & Catsup**
TUESDAY	Breakfast	**Grits**	6–8 olives	raw tomato	**Whole Wheat Zwieback**	**Bean Gravy**
	Dinner	**Sunflower Loaf**	**Baked Okra & Tomato**	bell peppers	**Tortillas**	
WEDNESDAY	Breakfast	**Grapenuts**	raisins on **Grapenuts**	**Orange Sauce**	**Boston Brown Bread**	**Sesame Butter**
	Dinner	**Lentils with Rice**	**Greens** with lemon juice	sliced tomatoes	**Buckwheat Crispies**	lemon juice
THURSDAY	Breakfast	rye waffles	blueberries/**Med. Sauce**	apple nut sauce		
	Dinner	**Paella Garbanzos**	**Baked Sweet Potatoes**	green salad with lemon	**Whole Wheat Crackers**	**Gravy**
FRIDAY	Breakfast	**Popcorn** (1–2 qts.)	fruit pudding	apple	**Toast**	
	Dinner	toasted nuts (¼ c.)	brussel sprouts	apple grated carrot salad	**Rye or Barley Bread**	
SABBATH	Breakfast	**Baked Millet**	pears	strawberries	**Corn-on-the-Cob**	**Soy Sour Cream** on Corn
	Dinner	**Pizza**	(veg. in **Main Dish**)	cucumber/lemon juice		avocado slices

Bold Print indicates items listed in the INDEX

SAMPLE MENUS

MEAL PLANNER

Regular Diet		Main Dish (Good in Protein and B-vitamins)	Second Dish	Raw Dish (Good in vitamin C)	Whole Grain Bread	Regular Diet — Spread, Nuts, Olives, or Avocado
SUNDAY	Breakfast	Corn Dodgers	Stewed Prunes	apples	Whole Wheat Toast	cashew cream
	Dinner	green peas and Potatoes in Cashew Gravy	String Beans	lettuce	Oatmeal Buns	
MONDAY	Breakfast	Pain Perdu	Blackberry Sauce	banana	Wheat Gems	Nut Butter
	Dinner	Hoppin' John	Beets in Lemon Juice	cauliflowerets	Pumpernickel	lemon juice
TUESDAY	Breakfast	Soy Waffles	Apple Butter	grapes	Tortillas	Carob Tahini Butter
	Dinner	Frijoles Con Chili	Squash Tamale Bake	celery strips	Barley Cakes	Agar Cheese
WEDNESDAY	Breakfast	corn fillets	Sautéed Breakfast Apple	orange	Doughnuts	Soy Spread
	Dinner	Mashed Split Peas	Kabobs	onion slices	Chapatis	Soy Sour Cream
THURSDAY	Breakfast	Rice Fritters	Fruit Sauce	pear	Apple Corn Bread	toasted nuts (2 T.)
	Dinner	Sprouted Lentils	Radishes in Cream	tomato quarters	Rye Bread	Nut Cheese
FRIDAY	Breakfast	Maranola	Orange Sauce	plums	Aerated Oatmeal Gems	Sesame Butter
	Dinner	Soy Cheese Balls	Stuffed Squash	sliced cucumbers	Melba Toast	Golden Sauce
SABBATH	Breakfast	French Toast	Queen Sauce	grapefruit	Gem Dandies	
	Dinner	Bean Puree	tomatoes, thickened	Cole Slaw	Spoon Bread	peanuts, toasted

Bold Print indicates items listed in the INDEX

XII. MENUS

SAMPLE MENUS

MEAL PLANNER

Spare Diet	Main Dish (Good in Protein and B-vitamins)	Second Dish	Raw Dish (Good in vitamin C)	Whole Grain Bread	Spare Diet — Spread, Nuts, Olives, or Avocado
SUNDAY Breakfast	oatmeal		**Fruit Sauce**	**Melba Toast**	almonds (4–5)
Dinner	**Paella**		sliced tomatoes	**Corn Dodgers**	olives (4)
MONDAY Breakfast	Rice Pudding		pear	crackers	**Nut Milk** (2 T.)
Dinner	**Baked Beans**	summer squash	celery sticks	**Oatmeal Buns**	**Wheatonnaise** / **Sunny Tomato Dressing**
TUESDAY Breakfast	**French Toast**		strawberry sauce		**Pecan Butter** (1 t.)
Dinner	Dry Rice	**Lentil & Tomato Soup**	carrot curls	**Corn Fritos**	avocado (½)
WEDNESDAY Breakfast	**Millet**		**Fruit Sauce**	**Melba Toast**	**Gravy** / **Wheatonnaise**
Dinner	**Split Pea Soup**	baked butternut squash	cucumbers	**Croutons**	lemon juice
THURSDAY Breakfast	baked oats		peaches on **Baked Oats**	**Popcorn**	carob nut milk (¼ c.)
Dinner	**Garbanzos, Mexican Style**	corn & okra	lettuce	**Baked Corn**	olives (4)
FRIDAY Breakfast	**Granola**		**Fruit Sauce**	**Melba Toast**	**Nut Milk**
Dinner	**Jamaica Peas**	zucchini	tomato	**Oatmeal Buns**	
SABBATH Breakfast	**Fruited Oats**		**Fruit Sauce**	**Corn Bread**	pumpkin seed (1 oz.)
Dinner	red bean puree	collards	bell peppers	**Corn Muffins**	**Soyonnaise**

Bold Print indicates items listed in the INDEX

SAMPLE MENUS

MEAL PLANNER

Spare Diet		Main Dish (Good in Protein and B-vitamins)	Second Dish	Raw Dish (Good in vitamin C)	Whole Grain Bread	Spread, Nuts, Olives, or Avocado
SUNDAY	Breakfast	Grits		apple	Rye Toast	Sesame Butter (1 t.)
	Dinner	Scalloped Potatoes	asparagus	grated carrots	Whole Wheat Bread	olives (4)
MONDAY	Breakfast	Cream of Wheat		Fruit Sauce	Melba Toast	almonds (4)
	Dinner	Calsoup or Ragout	Potatoes in jackets	Cole Slaw	crackers	nuts (2T.)
TUESDAY	Breakfast	Baked Grits		grapes	Whole Wheat Toast	Cashew Gravy (2 T.)
	Dinner	Millet Loaf	English peas	sliced tomatoes	Hush Puppies	Seasoned Gravy (2 T.)
WEDNESDAY	Breakfast	Corn Meal Soufflé		apple	Popcorn	Nut Cream
	Dinner	Shepherd Pie		onion slices	Whole Wheat Bread	olives (4)
THURSDAY	Breakfast	Oat Waffle	stewed apricots	plum	Carrot Corn Bread	Apple Butter
	Dinner	Lentil Pot	Cabbage	shredded carrots		olives (4)
FRIDAY	Breakfast	Swedish Farina		apple	Melba Toast	Soy Sour Cream (1 T.)
	Dinner	Oat Burgers		Alfalfa Sprouts	burger buns	Mustard & Catsup
SABBATH	Breakfast	Auf Lauf		Peaches	Corn Bread	Nut Dressing
	Dinner	Tostados		chopped lettuce and tomatoes	Tostados or Croutons	

Bold Print indicates items listed in the INDEX

XII. MENUS

SAMPLE MENUS

MEAL PLANNER

Fat Free Diet	Main Dish (Good in Protein and B-vitamins)	Second Dish	Raw Dish (Good in vitamin C)	Whole Grain Bread	Fat Free Diet — Spread, Nuts, Olives, or Avocados
SUNDAY Breakfast	oatmeal	raisins	apple	Zwieback	Apple Butter
Dinner	Garbanzos	Stuffed Peppers	Cole Slaw	Gem Dandies	
MONDAY Breakfast	Corn Waffles	Apple Butter	blueberries	Corn Pones	
Dinner	Holiday Roast	Corn-on-the-Cob	Tomato Aspic		
TUESDAY Breakfast	Auf Lauf	Fruit Sauce	orange	toast	fruit butter
Dinner	Chow Mein	Mashed Potatoes	Potato Salad	Wheat Gems	
WEDNESDAY Breakfast	French Toast	stewed fruit	banana	Oatmeal Buns	Dessert Topping
Dinner	Pea Patties	Thickened Tomatoes	Tebula		
THURSDAY Breakfast	Maranola	Apricot Sauce	grapefruit	Baked Millet	
Dinner	Sunflower Loaf	Georgia Gumbo	Golden Slaw	Corn Fritters	
FRIDAY Breakfast	Prune Cake		pears	toast	fruit butter
Dinner	Eggplant Patties	field peas	onion slices	hamburger buns	Soy Spread
SABBATH Breakfast	Arkansas Puddin'	steamed okra	fresh pineapple	Zwieback	Applesauce
Dinner	Lima Bean Casserole		tomato-lettuce salad	Corn Bread	

Bold Print indicates items listed in the INDEX

SAMPLE MENUS

MEAL PLANNER

Fat Free Diet

Day		Main Dish (Good in Protein and B-vitamins)	Second Dish	Raw Dish (Good in vitamin C)	Whole Grain Bread	Spread, Nuts, Olives, or Avocado
SUNDAY	Breakfast	Berry Pie	Applesauce	orange	Zwieback	
	Dinner	Split Pea Casserole	Broccoli	carrot curls	Oat Dodgers	
MONDAY	Breakfast	Banana Cream Toast		strawberries	Croutons	
	Dinner	Corn Tamale Pie	Zucchini	bell peppers	Zwieback	
TUESDAY	Breakfast	Apple Crisp	Applesauce	grapes	toast	Soy Spread
	Dinner	baked potatoes	String Beans	sliced tomatoes	dinner rolls	
WEDNESDAY	Breakfast	Oat Dodgers	Orange Sauce	blackberries		
	Dinner	Scalloped Eggplant	Dinner Carrots	lettuce wedges	Corn Muffins	
THURSDAY	Breakfast	"Cream of Rice"	Applesauce	mango	Zwieback Fingers	
	Dinner	Millet Loaf	Cream of "Mushroom" Soup	tomato wedges	Baked Millet	
FRIDAY	Breakfast	"All Bran"	raisins	blueberries		Dessert Topping
	Dinner	Chili Grits	Jerusalem Artichokes	cucumber salad	Croutons	
SABBATH	Breakfast	Banana Cream Pie		tangerine	Melba Toast	
	Dinner	Lentil Pot	squash	raw vegetable dish	Cereal Fillets	

Bold Print indicates items listed in the INDEX

XII. MENUS

PRIMARY RULES OF NUTRITION

1. Use a wide variety of foods during the year.
2. Keep individual meals simple: two or three dishes with bread and spread.
3. The **Essential Four Food Groups** provide all nutritive elements we need: vegetables, fruits, whole grains, and nuts.
4. Eat a **Balanced Diet**, not "high" in any food element, such as "a high protein diet" or "a high fat diet."
5. Use concentrated foods sparingly. It is advised that one not exceed $1/2$–1 teaspoon of salt daily or 3–5 teaspoons of sugar.
6. Do not serve fruits and vegetables at the same meal. Do not serve large amounts of liquid foods, or provide beverages to "wash the food down."
7. Foods should be cooked a proper length. Most foods require little cooking, but grains, legumes, and coarse vegetables require long cooking, often several hours.
8. Have a set mealtime with a minimum of 5–6 hours between meals.
9. Allow no between meals eating, not even an apple (or its juice).
10. Chew all food to a cream in the mouth. The benefit and the satisfaction from food depend much on the length of time it spends in the mouth.

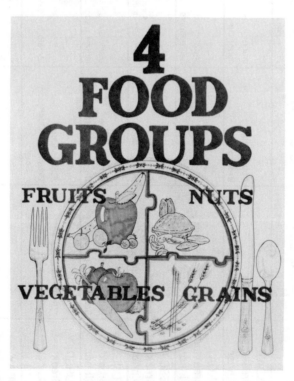

Essential Four Food Groups

Bold Print indicates items listed in the INDEX

XIII. CANNING DRYING SOAPMAKING

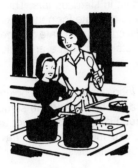

PRINCIPLES OF CANNING
_____

All kinds of fruit and most vegetables can be preserved in glass jars by methods easily applied in the home. There are two methods commonly used.

The **Hot-Pack or Open-Kettle Method,** consists of cooking the foods in a kettle either in their own juice or in water, then packing and sealing them in sterilized jars. This method is successful for acid fruits and acid vegetables, but is not adequate for nonacid products, such as corn, peas, beans, etc., as it is much more difficult to eliminate the germ that causes **Botulism** in nonacid foods. It is also difficult to retain the shape and color of the products canned in this way.

The **Cold-Pack Method** consists of packing uncooked foods in jars, then cooking them in the closed jars. All foods do not need to be and should not be cooked the same length of time. Herein the **Cold-Pack Method** is most successful. Foods are sterilized, and their flavor and color best retained, when definite timetables are followed, which have been developed after much experimenting. There are six steps as follows:

1. PREPARATION: The foods are cleaned, pitted, peeled, or sliced, to make them more attractive, and to avoid preserving useless material.

2. BLANCHING: This means to parboil, or scald a given length of time, which varies from 1–15 minutes, depending on the kind of product. For berries and soft fruits, the blanching is omitted. After washing the fruit or vegetables in cold water drop into boiling water for the required length of time, counting the time after boiling begins again.

3. COLD DIP: Lift the vegetables or fruit from the boiling water, and immediately plunge into cold water, lift, and drain. This cold dip sets the color and shrinks the food after it has been in the boiling water.

4. PACKING: The product should be immediately packed in hot jars which have been heated in the oven at 210° for 10 minutes. For fruits, hot juice, or water is added. For vegetables, hot water is added unless they are juicy. Fruit of any kind suitable for canning may be preserved without sugar. The sugar can be added when the fruit is used, exactly as is done with fresh fruit. If the fruit when canned is thoroughly ripe, it may be eaten without any additional sugar, and is sweet enough for most. The riper the fruit, provided it is sound, the more natural sugar, flavor, and nutrients it contains.

5. HOT-WATER BATH: The filled jars are set in a kettle or canner containing warm water. There will be less breakage of jars if the water bath is not boiling when jars are added. Hot water must reach at least to top of the food level in the jars, and may cover jars by 1″.

6. PROCESSING: The time is counted from the moment the water boils up well. As soon as the time is up, the jars are removed, set on a deck to cool, separated by at least 1″.

Steam Pressure Canner: Follow the directions for the HOT-WATER BATH method except that the water level is not up to the top of the food in the jars. Use only 2 quarts of water in the canner. Follow the timetable given on the following page.

Canning in Quart Jars

	Blanching before canning or freezing	Hot-Water Bath	10 Pounds Pressure
Vegetables (no salt needed)	Minutes	Hours	Minutes
Sweet corn	5	3	85
Green peas	2	3	40
Lima beans	5	3	50
String beans	2	3	25
Okra	2	2	40
Greens	15	3	90
Pumpkin	5	3	60
Tomatoes	1–2	$3/4$	15
Sweet potatoes	10	3	90
			5 Pounds Pressure
Fruits (no sugar needed)			
Apples	5	$1/4$	5
Pears	5–10	$1/4$	5
Quinces	5–10	$1/4$	5
Apricots	Raw Pack	$1/2$	10
Peaches	Raw Pack	$1/2$	10
Plums	$1/2$	$1/4$	8
Berries	Raw Pack	$1/4$	8

Botulism

The botulinus toxin is a heat labile protein which can be destroyed by boiling for at least 15 minutes. It is an exotoxin produced by the anaerobic growth of **Clostridium Botulinum,** in under processed, nonacid canned foods. The foods usually responsible for this type of food poisoning are meats, fish, and vegetables. Olives and fruits are rarely responsible. Less than 1 teaspoon of contaminated food can be fatal. The symptoms are nausea and vomiting with abdominal distress. Double vision and muscular paralysis are regular symptoms. Slurred speech and difficulty swallowing are also the usual. Fifty per cent of affected persons die. It can be prevented by boiling for 15 minutes any food suspected of contamination.

Bold Print indicates items listed in the INDEX

CANNING SPECIAL FOODS
_____

Canned Campmeeting Wheat

1¹/₄ c. whole kernel wheat

Place washed wheat in a quart jar. Fill to shoulder of jar with water. Process for 1 hour at 5–10 pounds pressure, or water bath for 3 hours. **Rice, Oat Groats, Barley,** or other whole grain may be processed similarly. It is now ready for heating at camp breakfast. Serve with a **Fruit Sauce.** May be used in any **Rice** is used, in stews or roasts.

Cucumber Relish

3 qts. sliced cucumbers   ¹/₂ c. salt
3 large onions

Let stand 4 hours. Drain, save liquid for **Soyonnaise** or cooking vegetables.

1 c. lemon juice   1 t. celery seed
1 c. water   3 bay leaves
1 c. honey

Boil the above five ingredients for 3 minutes. Add cucumber mixture and boil for 10 minutes very slowly. Dip into jars and seal. Green tomatoes may be substituted for cucumbers in this recipe to make **Green Tomato Relish.**

Dill Pickles

1 bay leaf   4 cloves garlic
1 grape leaf   1 head dill

Place the above four ingredients in the bottom of a jar. Pack whole or vertically sliced cucumbers in quart jar. Add 1¹/₂ tablespoons lemon juice, 1 tablespoon salt, one more head of dill and a grape leaf. Fill jar with boiling water and seal. Process in water bath canner 15 minutes.

Dried Beans, Peas, or Peanuts

1³/₄ c. dried legumes

Place washed, sorted legumes in a quart jar. Fill to shoulder of jar with water. Process for 1 hour at 10 pounds pressure. Boiled peanuts are especially fine prepared in this manner. When salted nicely and served over **Creamy Rice, Boiled Peanuts** make a very fine **Main Dish.**

Bold Print indicates items listed in the INDEX

Canned Nuts

4 c. nuts, raw

Place nuts in perfectly dry quart jar. Place cap. Process at 5 pounds pressure for 10 minutes, or water bath for 45 minutes. If salted nuts are preferred, coat nuts with 2 tablespoons oil to which $1/2$ teaspoon salt has been added. Increase processing time to 30 minutes at 5 pounds.

Fruits and Vegetables

Consult charts in common use if more detail is needed.

Canned Tomatoes with Fresh-ripe Flavor
Process Developed at Auburn University

1. Select firm-ripe tomatoes without green shoulders.
2. Wash in mild detergent solution and rinse well.
3. Scald in boiling water for 15 seconds.
4. Cool in running water and peel.
5. Slice with sharp knife about $3/8''$ thick.
6. Dip slices for 5 minutes in a 5% solution of calcium chloride. Put 1 cup powdered calcium chloride obtained from feed stores or druggist in 6 quarts of lukewarm water to make the 5% solution. This amount of solution will be enough for dipping one bushel of tomatoes.
7. Pack slices carefully in pint jars containing $1/4$ cup hot water, $1/2$ teaspoon salt, $1/2$ teaspoon sugar, and 1–2 tablespoons of lemon juice.
8. Fill jars with boiling water to within $1/2''$ of the top, seal loosely.
9. Heat in a boiling water bath for 10 minutes (15 minutes for quarts). Remove and tighten jar lids. Allow a few minutes of slow cooling.
10. Cool rapidly after danger of breaking jars is past in either running water or air stream. Refrigerate at least 24 hours, then store in a cool storage area up to one year.

Storage of Canned and Dried Foods: Vitamin losses during storage will increase if jars are stored at a temperature above 70°. Vitamin C and thiamine will be lost at a rate of 25% or more if stored at 80° for one year. The loss will be less than 15% if storage temperature is below 65°. Vitamin A and riboflavin are quite stable.

The process of drying does not cause major losses in vitamin content. When dried foods are stored in air, however, losses of vitamins A, C, and E may occur from reaction with oxygen. Store dried foods in tightly closed containers, preferably in a cold place.

Bold Print indicates items listed in the INDEX

ADVANTAGES OF DRYING FOODS

When foods are plentiful in season and the price is low, one can purchase at a fraction of the cost the same foods which will be bought dearly when out of season. If the foods have been produced in the home garden or orchard, the quality of the food can be known by the consumer. Commercially obtained foods may be packaged under conditions that the consumer would not allow if he were aware. The food may be under or over ripe, heat or cold damaged, or exposed to conditions of wilting or chemical fumes that might cause the consumer to reject the food. Drying food which has been personally inspected by the consumer can have a great appeal for its aesthetic factors.

Drying foods removes bulky water content, allowing storage in much less space than canned foods or fresh storage. The flavor of dried foods is sometimes even more appealing than in the fresh food. Few things are more satisfying than to follow a food from the planting of the seed to the eating of the food, especially if shared with dear friends who appreciate care taken to insure that everything has been done that can be done to develop excellence of nutritive value and safety of the product.

Drying Herbs

Cut herbs when the foliage is full, but before they bloom. Tie in bunches, label, and hang in a dry place, free from dust but where air circulates. When leaves are dry and will crumble, pick them from stems and store in labeled jars with tight fitting lids.

Herbs which yield seed should be harvested after full maturity has developed, but just before seed start to drop from seed pods. Place the seed pods on flat pans to dry. Thresh the seed and winnow to remove trash from the seed pods. Store seed in glass jars with tight fitting lids. Many seeds are suitable. Try dill, fennel, and coriander.

Drying Corn

Cut sweet corn from the cob and spread thinly on large flat pans lined with absorbent paper or sheets or cotton cloth. Cover pans with clean sheets and set in full sun. Stir often. Take inside at night. Primary drying should be finished in about 2 days. Pour the corn into clean white, cotton sacks. Hang up for 3 days in a warm, dry place to complete drying. Store in plastic bags or glass jars with tight lids. To prepare for table, soak overnight in water, add salt and simmer for 1 hour. Serve with **Margarine** or **Soy Sour Cream.** One cup dried corn serves 4–6.

Fresh Storage

Onions may be stored in a dry place by tying the tops securely in bundles and hanging the bundles in the pantry or a cool, dry place. Winter squash will store with no special care by keeping them in a cool, dry place. Many foods such as "sand pears," apples, sweet potatoes, eggplant, and many others can be best stored by wrapping each piece in paper and carefully placing in a barrel or box which is set in a cool, dry place. Check occasionally to insure against spoilage.

Leather Britches
Green Beans

Harvest tender beans and string them on a heavy white thread using a large eye needle. Hang the strings of beans in full sun. Take inside at night. Primary drying is finished in 2–3 days. Slide beans off the threads. Place on large flat pans in oven preheated for 5 minutes at 250°. As soon as the pans are placed in oven, turn oven off. Let pans remain in oven for 5 minutes. Remove, cool, store in tightly covered glass jars. To cook, break into small pieces and cover with water. Soak overnight. Boil for 4–6 hours, or pressure cook at 10 pounds for 1–1$\frac{1}{2}$ hours.

Drying Fruit

Apples, pears, peaches, bananas, and many other fruit may be easily dried on tables set in the sun by following simple directions. Good "drying ovens" can be improvised as follows: roll car windows up to 1" from top; use the greenhouse in summer; set an old refrigerator or stove in the sun and rig it for ventilation; a special cabinet designed for drying.

1. Select ripe, good quality fruit. Drying will not convert poor fruit into sweet, good tasting fruit.

2. Wash well. Peel apples and bananas. The skins may be left on many fruits such as peaches, pears, apricots, and plums.

3. Slice apples and sand pears in eighths. Bartlett pears, peaches, and apricots can be dried successfully when halved. Bananas should be quartered lengthwise. Figs and many small fruit may be left whole. Lay slices on large flat pans and set in full sun. Turn slices after 2–3 hours and occasionally during the next 2 or 3 days.

4. In case of rain, take fruit inside and complete the process in oven set at about 140°. If preferred, the whole drying process may be accomplished in the oven as follows: place pans of fruit in oven preheated to 250°. Reduce heat immediately to 140°. After 5 minutes, open oven door about 1–2" to allow escape of moisture. Thin slices require 6–10 hours. Pans of corn require 12–18 hours.

5. When fruit is well dried, store in plastic bags tied securely, or in glass jars with tight fitting lids.

6. Try your hand at drying unusual vegetables such as green peppers, pumpkin, root vegetables, or others. You will find it high adventure.

Bold Print indicates items listed in the INDEX

Lye Soap

6 c. water   5–6 lbs. oil **or** other fat
1 can lye

Boil the water and lye together until the lye is dissolved. Add the fat while boiling and stirring. Continue boiling after adding fat while stirring constantly for 20 minutes. Continue to simmer for another 30 minutes. Stir again and pour out into a shallow pan to harden. Cut into squares to harden.

Wood Lye

If you wish to make your own lye, place a bushel of hardwood ashes in a leaky wooden bucket, a hollow log, or other wood frame to hold the ashes. If needed, place paper, shucks, or straw in the bottom of the wooden container to filter the ashes. Pour water over the ashes. Collect one gallon of drippings from the ashes. To this amount of drippings, use about 10 pounds of fat. Boil and stir as directed under **Lye Soap.** The drippings contain both the water and the lye listed in the directions for **Lye Soap.**

Bold Print indicates items listed in the INDEX

XIV. KITCHEN TIPS

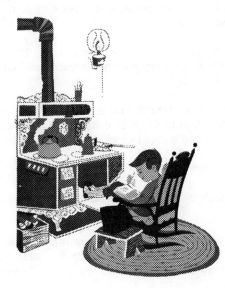

XIV. KITCHEN TIPS

1. Minimize nutrient losses from the deteriorating action of enzymes which work in the temperature range of 60° to 90° by starting vegetables in boiling water. These enzymes are denatured by boiling.

2. Long cooking of dry beans and grains reduces their gas forming potential. Also, use small servings, tiny bites, and long chewing on such gas formers as beans, apples, onions, bell pepper, etc.

3. Well cooked **Garbanzos** will take the place of meats and meat substitutes or nuts in most recipes without loss of flavor or consistency. The nutrition of the dish may actually improve by the use of this biologically superior bean.

4. When dry, 1 cup of beans represents $2^{1}/_{2}$ cups cooked.

5. Have a vegetable stock jar in the refrigerator to pour all liquid drained from vegetables.

6. "White" Karo syrup is less expensive and more readily available in some localities than honey and can be used interchangeably with it. It is not quite as sweet as honey volume for volume. Furthermore, acid fruits are not easily sweetened with Karo.

7. The fruits and vegetables in season are usually the most nourishing, and possibly the best able to supply the particular needs of the body during their season of the year.

8. To make **Flaky Rice,** stir only once at the beginning. To make **Creamy Rice,** stir occasionally during cooking and well at the end of the cooking time, using more water than for **Flaky Rice.**

9. Avoid cooking food that can yield as much flavor and nutritive value raw as cooked. Remember that some foods actually yield more nutrients after cooking. These include the root vegetables, legumes, and grains. Several legumes contain a toxin which can be destroyed by adequate cooking. Several varieties of soybeans contain this toxin.

10. Serve fresh parsley, fennel tops, or fennel or dill seed after garlic or onions to prevent garlic or onion breath.

11. Additional leavening action in breads and soufflés will be given by flours made from garbanzos, soybeans, lima beans, oats, rice, or sesame seed. **Soaked Soybeans** whirled in blender with an equal quantity of water until smooth serves the same purpose.

12. Use **Alfalfa Sprouts** in sandwiches instead of lettuce, as lettuce wilts more quickly.

13. The kernels of **Popcorn** that fail to pop can be ground into powder and added to cereals.

Bold Print indicates items listed in the INDEX

XIV. KITCHEN TIPS

14. In bread or roast recipes that call for eggs, use $1/4$ cup of fruit pulp for each egg. Prepare pulp by soaking and cooking 1 pound of dried fruit in 1 quart of water until tender. Liquefy in blender with 1 cup of cooking water and $1/3$ cup starch or tapioca. Store in the refrigerator and use when needed. Keep up to three weeks.

15. An oven temperature of 25° less should be used for glass baking dishes. If recipe states 350° for metal pans, use 325° for glass.

16. You can keep a variety of breads in the freezer to avoid monotony and eliminate stale breads. Bake extra waffles when you make waffles. Package and freeze the extra. Heat unthawed in a toaster or on a cookie sheet. Frozen waffles will keep many weeks.

17. When wheat flour or starch is used for sauce or any thickened dish which is to be stored frozen, when thawed and reheated it will curdle. This feature may be overcome by using rice flour instead. Rice flour may be purchased at any specialty food shop, or ground in a seed mill.

18. **Natural Insecticides:**

    a. Mosquitos: a spray of sesame oil.
    b. Ants: a bit of honey with 20 Mule Team borax powder.
    c. Roaches: a paste of powdered boric acid plus sweetened condensed milk.

19. **Electric Range Tips:**

    Your electric range cooks best when it is used correctly. Here are tips on how to get top efficiency from it.

    a. Use flat-bottom pans that fit the cooking element you're using. This reduces wasted heat and cooking time.
    b. Cook in the oven as much as you can. Since an electric range oven is thermostatically controlled, it is on only about $1/3$ of each hour it is used. Whenever possible, cook several foods in the oven at the same time.
    c. Use the oven for cooking food, not for heating the kitchen. A small electric heater does a more efficient job.
    d. Don't use the oven to toast bread; the toaster is much more efficient.
    e. Avoid opening the oven door until the food is cooked. Each time you open the door, 20% of the heat escapes. This can also cause improper browning and even baking failure.
    f. Turn off the oven and surface elements a few minutes, about five, before the food is cooked. The residual heat will finish the job.
    g. It takes a lot of energy to heat water. Use as little as possible to cook foods.
    h. When food boils, reduce the heat to low. The food will cook just as fast, but with less electricity.
    i. Keep pots and pans bright and shiny. This allows food to cook faster.
    i. Tight-fitting lids on pots and pans make cooking faster and keep the kitchen cooler. Remove the lids as infrequently as possible.

XV. INDEX

S

W

Y

Z

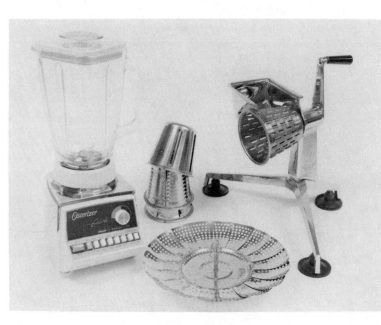

Food Preparation

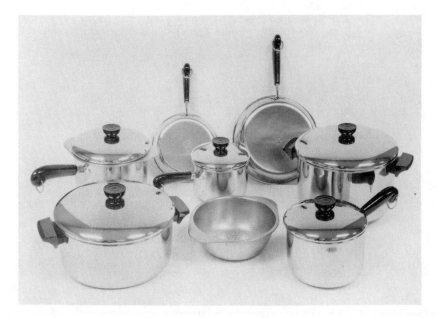

Select a Good Set of Cookware

Yuchi Pines Health Conditioning Center

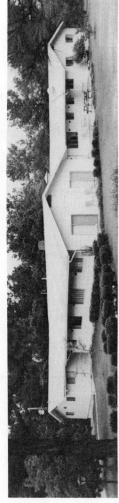

Your body knows naturally what it needs to stay healthy. And it tries to tell you...but have you been listening?

Most of us eat and drink too much, eat the wrong kinds of foods, drink beverages that are hard on body systems, exercise frantically and then feel worse rather than better. We can't relax when we "rest." We ignore the natural rhythms and requests of our bodies — and we get sick as a result.

But we can eat healthful foods prepared in healthful ways, drink the refreshing drinks nature provides, exercise through purposeful labor that is more beneficial than frantic "recreation." We can rest in natural tranquility. If we learn these simple skills, we stay healthy — really healthy....

Or we get well if we're sick.

Anvwodi (ah-niv-wo-di), the Cherokee word for "get well place," is the health conditioning center at Yuchi Pines. Here you learn to keep yourself in good health through use of nature's most powerful "drugs": pure air, sunlight, temperance, rest, spiritual support, exercise, proper diet, and that beneficent liquid — water. You become whole again while enjoying the peace and serenity of 200 acres of pine and oak woodland.

You'll have your own program of specially prescribed conditioning treatments. When you arrive you'll be given a physical examination and a laboratory analysis. Based on the results and a comprehensive medical interview you'll be given a program of rest, activity, diet, demonstrations, lectures, and natural therapy to bring you toward the peak of good health.

And of course, your physical and medical needs will be constantly monitored.

You'll eat fresh and delicious meals of homegrown fruits and vegetables, homemade cereals and natural breads — and learn how to prepare such healthful meals for yourself.

You'll breathe in life-restoring, pollution-free air and drink up Southern sunlight while gardening, hiking, chopping wood, or tending the orchard — the kind of labor that feels good because you're putting your muscles to healthy use.

You'll learn to use water to greatest advantage — to drink, to stimulate, to soothe.

You may choose to seek the warmth of family worship. You can elect this experience at Anvwodi. And if you wish, one of our chaplains will listen and discuss your spiritual concerns.

When you go home, how will you feel? If you continue the good, healthful habits you've learned at Yuchi Pines, you'll continue to feel as if you were still in the beautiful Alabama woodland, living a clean, simple, invigorating life.

What we're offering you is a lifetime of better living...as the Creator intended.

☐ YES, please send me more information about how I can condition myself for better living at Yuchi Pines Institute.

☐ I'd like to talk with someone about the health conditioning program.

My telephone number is ( )

Name

and Street

City _____ State _____ Apt. _____

Zip _____

Yuchi Pines Health Conditioning Center
Route 1, Box 273
Seale, Alabama 36875
Phone: 205/855-4764

OTHER BOOKS BY DR. THRASH

Home Remedies --9.95

The complete "how-to", listing 67 diseases and their remedies--from arthritis to whooping cough. Specializes in water (or hydro-) therapy. Also massage, charcoal, garlic, and other herbal therapies. "Treatments rely heavily on physiological processes that use the body's own defense mechanisms." --Baton Rouge Sun

Nutrition for Vegetarians --9.95

"The book speaks to adults as adults...which should help the reader gain a better understanding of vegetarianism, indeed, any diet." --L.A. Times

Eat for Strength Cookbook (Regular or Oil Free) --7.95

A delightful cookbook for those interested in cutting animal products, cholesterol, fat, and calories! "...a valuable cookbook." --L.A. Times

More Natural Remedies --6.95

Practical guide to treating many common illnesses. Designed to be read by professional and lay person alike. "...Genuine help for those seeking alternative...treatment." --Journal/Post

Food Allergies Made Simple --4.95

Parade magazine says food intolerance is involved in as much as 60% of all human illness. You owe it to yourself to have this book on hand.

The Animal Connection --4.95

According to the Department of Agriculture, there is no fowl or livestock anywhere that can be guaranteed disease-free. Pets also can be carriers of lethal ailments. Find out how to protect yourself.

P.M.S. : Premenstrual Syndrome --2.95

Conservatively, over 12 million American women suffer from P.M.S. Do you really know what it is? What to do about the problem is covered in this small, but comprehensive book.

Order Form

Name_____

Address_____

City_____ST_____

Zip_____

Postage and Handling:
U.S.--15% of order. Others--20%
Orders under $10.00 add $1.50 Handling Fee

Send orders to: NewLifestyle Books
                  Seale, AL 36875
                  (205) 855-4708

Prices subject to change
Pay in U.S. funds only.

____Nutrition for Veg. 9.95   ____
____Home Remedies 9.95   ____
____Eat for Strength 7.95   ____
____Oil-Free edition 7.95   ____
____More Natural Remedies 6.95 ____
____Animal Connection 4.95   ____
____Food Allergies 4.95   ____
____P.M.S. 2.95   ____
                                ____
                                ____
                                ____

Shipping and Handling   ____
Sales Tax 4% (AL only)   ____

Total Amount Enclosed   ____